Managing Health Promotion

ABOUT THE AUTHOR

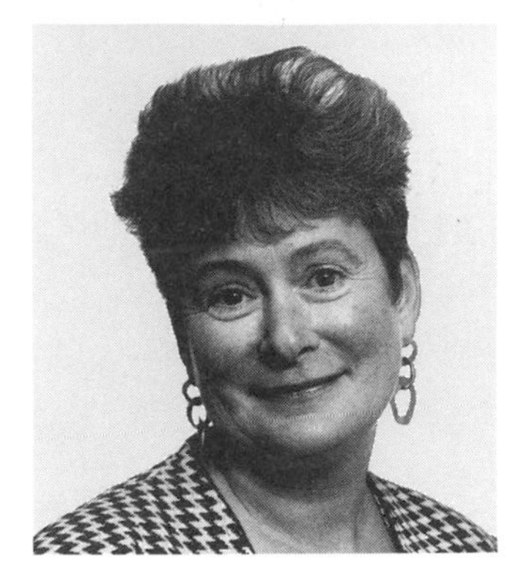

Ina Simnett MA (Oxon) DPhil CertEd

Dr Ina Simnett works as a Senior Research Fellow at Keele University, England, and as a freelance trainer and health promotion consultant. Her recent activities include coordinating and contributing to a project to generate learning materials for managers in the National Health Service who are designing and implementing the new UK strategy for health (the *Managing Health Improvement Project*, jointly commissioned by the Health Education Authority and the NHS Training Division and based in the Education Department, Keele University). She has also recently contributed to research and development work on *Interventions and Alliances to Promote Physical Activity* (also commissioned by the Health Education Authority and based in the Centre for Health Planning and Management, Keele University).

She was previously a writer and consultant for the *Certificate in Health Education Open Learning Project* (CHEOLP) at Keele University and also managed an Open Learning Centre for health service managers participating in the "*Managing Health Services*" open learning programme in the southwest of England (organized nationally by the Institute of Health Services Management). She has contributed to a number of open learning and training materials in health promotion.

She started her career as a research physiologist, then worked in health education for 12 years, including managing the Northumberland Health Education Department for five years, and coordinating a Health Education Authority alcohol education programme for southwest England. Later she worked as a training consultant with the National Health Service Training Authority, and as district training manager for Frenchay Health Authority in Bristol. She has extensive experience of planning and teaching health promotion to health professionals, teachers, social services staff and NHS managers in the UK, and to senior managers from health services in developing countries on the MBA (Health, Population and Nutrition Programme) in the Centre for Health Planning and Management, Keele University. She contributes to national conferences, and has recently undertaken health promotion consultancy in Australia.

She is the co-author of *Promoting Health: A Practical Guide*, the leading textbook on health promotion worldwide (Ewles, L. and Simnett, I., 1st edn, 1985, Chichester: Wiley; 2nd edn, 1992, London: Scutari Press; 3rd edn, 1995).

INA SIMNETT
MA (Oxon) DPhil
CertEd
Centre for Health Planning and Management, Keele University

Managing Health Promotion:

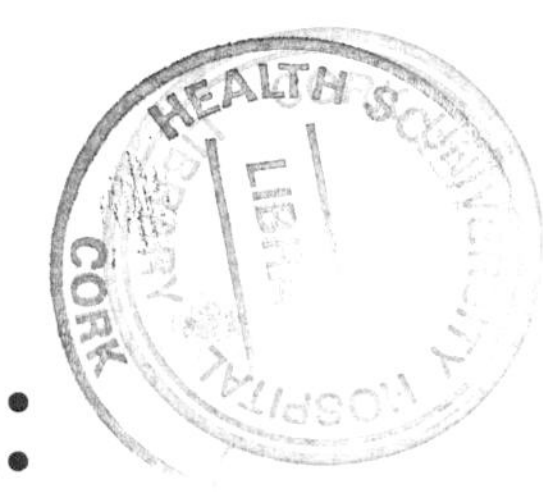

Developing Healthy Organizations and Communities

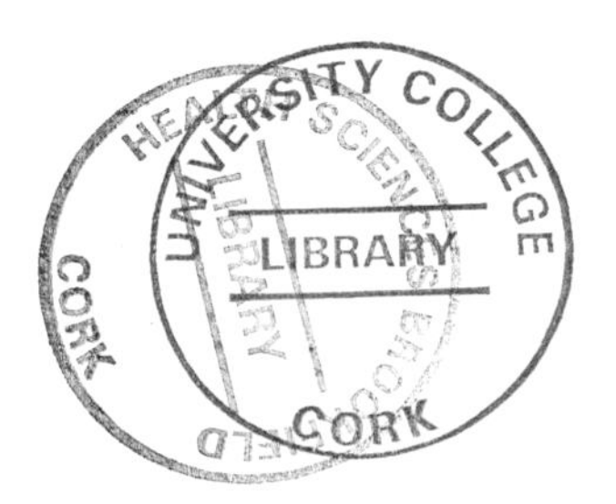

JOHN WILEY & SONS
Chichester · New York · Brisbane · Toronto · Singapore

Baffins Lane, Chichester.
West Sussex PO19 1UD, England

Telephone: National 01243 779777
International (+44) 1243 779777

Reprinted January 1996, January 1997, January 2001

Other Wiley Editorial Offices

John Wiley & Sons, Inc., 605 Third Avenue,
New York, NY 10158-0012, USA

Jacaranda Wiley Ltd, 33 Park Road, Milton,
Queensland 4064, Australia

John Wiley & Sons (Canada) Ltd, 22 Worcester Road,
Rexdale, Ontario M9W 1L1, Canada

John Wiley & Sons (SEA) Pte Ltd, 37 Jalan Pemimpin #05–04,
Block B, Union Industrial Building, Singapore 2057

British Library Cataloguing in Publication Data

A catalogue record for this book is available from the British Library

ISBN 0-471-95814-X

Typeset in 11/13 Palacio by Mathematical Composition Setters Ltd, Salisbury, England
Printed and bound in Great Britain by Redwood Books, Trowbridge, Wiltshire

This book is printed on acid-free paper responsibly manufactured from sustainable forestation, for which at least two trees are planted for each one used for paper production.

To all those managers and
workers willing to invest in
developing organizations
which contribute towards
better health and well-being

CONTENTS

FOREWORD

A decade ago an important new book appeared in the field of health promotion, co-authored by Ina Simnett and Linda Ewles, offering a practical guide for all those who practised health promotion in their everyday work. Its value was quickly recognized, and demonstrated by the frequency with which it has been reprinted subsequently, and is now in its third edition.

Anything that is labelled "practical" runs the risk of being considered rather ephemeral and lacking in rigour. As readers of the Simnett and Ewles text discovered, they had avoided that accusation by delivering a text that was both demanding of the reader yet readable and full of good ideas.

It's hardly a surprise, therefore, to find people eagerly awaiting the latest text to appear from one of the same authors, Ina Simnett. This time, attention is directed at managers and managing for better health—but, again as an essentially practical guide with a familiar (user-friendly) format, with plenty of examples, checklists, notes and references and, above all, good sense throughout.

Yes, the text does offer models and frameworks, concepts and techniques; and, again, these are translated into good advice and illustrations so that lessons can be learnt. Thus, for instance, the reader can turn to the text as a source reference to grasp the meaning of such terms as: health promotion, health gain, competence-based assessment, quality circles, audit, healthy alliances, leadership attributes, life cycles, empowerment, and so on.

Equally, clear and unambiguous guidance is offered on a variety of agendas in the management field, including: designing a health development strategy; developing the health potential of your staff; mapping the health promotion role, and how to specify quality; how to conduct a health promotion audit; how to set goals and objectives for health promotion; how to reduce conflict and improve the quality of working life; and how to develop health-promoting workplaces.

The final passage of the book is subtitled "Reaching the Parts and People that Others Miss". In many ways, this captures quite neatly the overall worth of this new book. If one had perfect foresight, one would be tempted to predict that this book would be a best-seller in its field; even without such a gift, one can be reasonably confident that it will be a winner, and deservedly so.

Kenneth Lee
Professor and Director,
Centre for Health Planning and Management,
Keele University, UK

PREFACE

This book is about management development, organizational development, professional development, personal development and leadership development for better health. It aims to provide a concise, practical and easy-to-read guide to the improved management of health promotion, and thence to contribute to improving the effectiveness and efficiency of health promotion work and to improving competence in the development of health-promoting people, organizations, partnerships and communities. I use the word management as meaning *the process of managing*. In this context, management is the collective (corporate) responsibility of everyone working within an organization, starting with the management board, including those designated as managers and all other staff. This book is therefore aimed at more than just managers, although they will have a particular interest in it. While it is written primarily for those who work in the National Health Service (NHS) in the United Kingdom of Great Britain and Northern Ireland (the UK), it is also suitable for those who work in other settings, whether they work in the public sector, for example as health managers working in environmental health services, or as managers or professionals working in social services, prisons, the police or schools; as workers in the voluntary sector, for example voluntary organizations or pressure groups; or those who work in the private sector, for example in private health care or social care services, leisure services or commercial businesses. Managers and professionals with a role in health promotion, working in other countries (both developed and developing), may also find the practical approach taken by this book helpful.

It is aimed at all those people, working within organizations, who have significant management responsibilities in their jobs (whether or not they have the title of "manager"), and who actually, or potentially, are responsible for managing health promotion work or for allocating resources for health development. These include managers and staff of specialist health promotion services, but these form only a small part of the "army" of managers and professionals working within both purchasing and providing agencies who have health promotion responsibilities. These are drawn from across the range of health, education and caring and other public sector professions, and include senior nurses, senior teachers, general practitioners (GPs), social work team leaders, environmental health officers, public health physicians, and members of the professions allied to medicine, in addition to general managers and business managers.

All businesses have a health promotion role related to the health and well-being of their staff, and this book will therefore be of interest to executives, managers, personnel officers and occupational health staff in commercial enterprises. It will be of especial interest to those businesses who are partners in health alliances, for example these related to the supply of healthy foods or the provision of health-enhancing services. Many voluntary agencies have a health promotion role, and this book will enable them to improve their management of health promotion activities, to compete for health promotion contracts, and to work together with other agencies. It is not, however, intended as a substitute for comprehensive management development and training, but seeks to raise awareness of the competencies required for meeting the challenges of health promotion. This book will also be of interest to tutors of health studies and social care studies, to tutors of health promotion and of health, education and social services management courses, to tutors of GP training courses, and to students on these courses. Those involved in research and development work related to health promotion will also find it useful. It may also be of interest to chief executives and non-executive directors on the boards of organizations, who wish to play a part in developing their organization as a health-promoting one.

Many of the activities we need to invest in for improving health through health promotion work can only be delivered through partnerships (health alliances) between organizations at local level. *Health alliances are two or more agencies working together to achieve health gain, which agencies working on their own could not achieve as effectively or efficiently.* Some health alliances will have a wholly health promotion focus; others will span across health promotion into other areas of health gain, such as diagnosing, treating and caring for people with particular health problems. Each of these agents and agencies will have their own unique objectives and areas of expertise. In order to work together, they need to identify *shared objectives,* many of which will focus on prevention/health promotion. This book will therefore be of interest to all those working within health alliances, or who are aiming to develop potential alliances.

The need for this book originates from three changes in the UK: the health service reforms initiated by the NHS and Community Care Act 1990; the development of a national strategy for health, as set out in the government White Paper *The Health of the Nation* (and corresponding documents for Scotland, Wales and Northern Ireland); and the implementation of the *Caring for People* White Paper, through providing vulnerable people with care in the community. Together these are having a major impact on health promotion, both on how it is managed and organized and on its place in the public "agenda". Managers and professionals within the NHS and beyond are now grappling with developing and implementing health strategies through managing major developments, such as expanding their field of health promotion work, introducing continuous quality management of health promotion work, developing their organization into a health-promoting one (through measures such as developing staff to work in autonomous teams), and developing health partnerships and ways of joint working with other agencies. All these developments must be managed, and managed well. We are not yet equipped to do this. The agenda for the management development, organizational development and personal development required is very large and will take time to realise. This book is one contribution to that agenda.

THE PURPOSE AND OBJECTIVES OF THE BOOK

The purpose of the book is to assist in improving the management and leadership of health promotion. It aims to be "down to earth" and succinct, but at the same time to avoid being superficial, through providing good signposting for those who wish to pursue particular subjects in more depth. Each chapter, therefore, ends with references and suggestions for further reading. The book also aims to help readers to reflect on and learn from their own experiences. I have therefore included suggestions for questions readers could ask themselves and activities to do as an individual or in a group.

It has the following specific objectives:

1. To raise awareness of the crucial importance of empowering people, in order to be effective in health promotion management, and of the skills and competencies this requires.
2. To enable managers and professionals to develop their organizations into "health-promoting organizations" which provide a role model for other organizations and indeed for how health promotion can be carried out across the whole community.
3. To provide managers and professionals with techniques and understanding which enable them to be powerful at health development: anticipating change, fostering health promotion innovations, adapting to new circumstances, modifying the environment to maintain their success, and coupling a vision, of health-promoting people, organizations, alliances and communities, to action.

4. To enable managers and professionals to continually improve health promotion work through designing and implementing strategies for continuous quality improvement.
5. To provide examples and case studies of how health promotion work is being managed, and how health-promoting organizations and partnerships are being developed, in order to spread good management practices.
6. To raise awareness of the key competencies required for the management of health promotion.
7. To enable managers and professionals to plan and evaluate their health promotion work, using the concept of health gain, and the health gain spiral, as the fundamental yardstick.
8. To enable managers and professionals to build health alliances and to improve their effectiveness at joint working aiming to promote better health.
9. To enable managers and professionals to take steps to assist local people in sharing control of health promotion.

The book on health promotion, which I co-authored with Linda Ewles,* has been highly acclaimed. It is aimed primarily at health promoters (all the professionals who practice face-to-face "health promotion" with their clients and patients). This book complements *Promoting Health*, through focusing on the management of health promotion by, for example, enhancing understanding of how to supervise and improve the performance of health promoters and through spreading good management practices. I do not, therefore, repeat much of the information in Ewles and Simnett, which is relevant to the management of health promotion, but provide extensive cross-references.

This book is largely based on research and development work which I carried out while working as the coordinator of the *Managing Health Improvement Project* (MAHIP), established in 1992 in the Department of Education of Keele University, with the brief to develop training materials in health promotion and health improvement for management staff in the health services in England. This project has been jointly commissioned by the Health Education Authority and the NHS Training Division. Further information about the project and the availability of the open learning materials it is producing can be obtained from the Health Education Authority.†

---

* Ewles, L. and Simnett, I. (3rd edn 1995) *Promoting Health: A Practical Guide*, London: Scutari Press.

†Professional Development, Health Education Authority, Hamilton House, Mabeldon Place, London WC1H 9TX. Tel: 0171 3833833.

ACKNOWLEDGEMENTS

In the preparation of this book, use has been made of ideas and suggestions which I, or other people, developed while I was working as coordinator of the *Managing Health Improvement Project* (MAHIP). The usefulness of these sources is gratefully acknowledged. Where ideas were generated by other people than myself, I have made every effort to identify these individuals in the text. I especially acknowledge the influence of Dr Peter Brambleby, Pat Dark, Pat Evans, Glenn MacDonald, Moira Bremner and Liz Rolls. Ben Totterdale, Ian Foster, Kate Lucy and Pat Mahoney also provided me with very useful advice and guidance. I also acknowledge the support of Geraldine Tibbs and Pauline Marshall of the Health Education Authority, and Sue Prosser, Nigel Cocks and Ian Bennett of the NHS Training Division, who commissioned MAHIP. I am deeply indebted to Professor Richard Kempa, director of MAHIP, and to members of the Project Advisory Committee, especially Marion Balcombe, Pat Faber, Richard Parish and Peter England (the Project Advisory Committee chairman), and to Sue Barnard, the project secretary.

While working on MAHIP, in the Department of Education at Keele University, I also spent some time working on another project, also commissioned by the Health Education Authority, and based in the Centre for Health Planning and Management at Keele University. This research project, "*Interventions and Alliances to Promote Physical Activity*", helped me to develop my ideas related to how best to work in partnerships for health. I am grateful for the unfailing support of my colleagues on this project, Dr Steve Cropper, Joyce Abbatt and Peter Folwell, and to Professor Kenneth Lee, Director of the Centre for Health Planning and Management, for the encouragement and support he gave me, to get on with writing this book.

I would like to acknowledge the influence of Dr John Øvretveit, who has made an enormous contribution to the health service in defining and describing quality and who helped me to develop my ideas about quality of health promotion. Dr Viv Speller similarly helped me to develop ideas about how to work effectively in "health alliances". I am especially grateful to those people who have contributed case material which hopefully enables the book to have "real-life" relevance: Liz Perkins, Peter Allen and Tony Williams of the Dorcan School. Many other people have influenced the content of this book, particularly managers in the health service and managers in specialist health promotion services. I am also very grateful for help I received related to the role of health-promoting hospitals, from Dominic Harrison and, related to Agenda 21, from Andrew Rogers. I wish to thank my colleagues and friends, Liz Rolls, Jenny Moon and Dr Margaret Sills, for our stimulating discussions, inspiring lunch, and for the contribution of much useful information and ideas. Thank you, also, to Rae Magowan, Terry Bell and Beryl Wardley, for enabling me to attend the Trent Health Promotion Audit Dissemination Day, on 10 November 1994.

Finally, I would like to thank Caroline Plaice and Sheila Headford, the wonderful library staff at Frenchay Postgraduate Medical Centre, and those people who have read draft material and offered me constructive comments: Joyce Abbatt, Elizabeth Williams, Linda Ewles and Peter England. I also thank my long-suffering husband, who had considerable difficulty sometimes in tearing me away from the word processor. Writing a book can sometimes be a lonely activity, and it was the discussions with my husband which spurred me on when the going was tough and ensured that the book was completed.

CHAPTER 1 What is health promotion and why invest in it?

Summary

The chapter starts by discussing what health promotion is. It asserts that there are two fundamental aspects to health promotion: the end result, which is improved health and well-being; and the means, which is enabling people and communities to take charge of aspects of their lives which affect their health. It continues by describing four main areas for investment in health promotion: the extension of services and policies which we know are effective; improving standards of living; improving the environment; and modifying lifestyles; and suggests some reasons organizations might have for investing in health promotion. It then discusses the concept of health gain and describes the health gain spiral as the yardstick for all organizations to use in managing their health promotion work. It discusses what is meant by health promotion management and highlights two key aspects of managing for success: working in health partnerships, and working within "health-promoting organizations". Finally, it emphasizes the importance of making links between the health and environment agendas. It ends with some questions you could ask yourself.

THE MEANING OF HEALTH PROMOTION

Many documents have been written about the meaning and purpose of health promotion, and it is not my intention to describe theoretical models of health promotion here. However, thinking about the meaning and purpose of what we do is important, before plunging into action, and suggestions for further reading are provided at the end of this chapter (1).

Basically, health promotion is an umbrella term for a very wide range of activities which enhance good health and well-being and prevent ill-health (2). It includes:

- Health education and health information.
- Preventive medical measures (such as screening clinics and immunization).

- Healthy public policies (such as regulations about smoking in public places).
- Environmental measures which improve health and safety (such as traffic calming and the provision of good, affordable housing).
- Community and organizational health development (enabling communities and organizations to identify and meet their needs for better health).

A fundamental characteristic of health promotion is that it aims to empower people to take increased control over aspects of their lives which affect their own, and others', health (3). This "empowerment" is not about enabling individuals to have power over other people, but is "mutual empowerment": about sharing power so that everyone gains health benefits. It is thus inextricably linked with concepts such as democracy, autonomy, community and participation. It is political, with a small "p", and focuses on how people can take increased responsibility for their own, and others', health. It is about forging relationships through which everyone gains improved self-esteem, and learns how best to live and work and play together for mutual advantage.

Naturally, government policies shape the wider environment. All the policies of government have an impact on health (for example, the distribution of wealth in society has a major influence on health). Here, however, we are primarily concerned with how managers working within organizations at local level can invest in health promotion, as part of, or in some instances, the whole of, their business. (In the case of managers of specialist health promotion services, for example, it is the whole of their business.) We are concerned with what can be done through health promotion activities to improve health by:

- Improving health education (through, for example, improved provisions by schools and educational institutions and in the workplace).
- Improving health and well-being (through, for example, better measures by social services, voluntary organizations and in the workplace).
- Creating conditions which enhance health and well-being (through, for example, town planning, environmental health services, better public transport, and leisure and recreation services).
- Improving health employment opportunities (for example, in commercial enterprises which play a part in enhancing health and well-being).

It is important to note that health promotion is not only a function of the professions working in health care services. It is a core function of all those professions and disciplines working in the health and social care sector, the education sector, the town and country planning sector, the sports and leisure sector, environmental health services, the transport sector, the police, the housing sector and many other settings. It therefore spans right across the public sector. It is also a key function for many of those working in the voluntary sector, who have key roles in advocacy and advice for particular groups in the population. It is a function of many businesses related to the "healthy" goods and services they provide, such as manufacturers of safe toys, sales of healthy foods, and commercial providers of health, sports, recreation and leisure facilities. All businesses have a health promotion function, insofar as they are all concerned with the health and well-being of their employees and with improving their work performance. All these workers and businesses require management of their health promotion activities and, in addition, need to have mutually empowering processes which provide a high quality of working life for everyone. This book is therefore about the processes of managing all the systems, structures, services, programmes, projects and people within organizations in order to optimize health and well-being. These management processes are a collective (corporate) responsibility not only of executives and managers, but of all those (such as doctors, senior nurses and many other occupations and professions) who are responsible for decisions which allocate resources to health and health promotion work.

Concepts and determinants of health and well-being

I use the phrase "health and well-being" to encompass all aspects of health and well-being. According to Doyal and Gough (4) well-being can be defined as "the ability of people to participate in life". In order for well-being to be achieved two basic needs must first be fulfilled: the need for *health* and the need for *autonomy* (autonomy means, literally, self-rule and from it are derived other moral principles such as individual liberty, the right of confidentiality and the right to privacy). Health promotion enables individuals, families, groups and communities to optimize their health and well-being whatever their needs or stage of development. It is thus anti-discriminatory and focuses on those aspects of health and well-being which are the current priorities for the individuals concerned. This could be social well-being, physical health, emotional health, intellectual health or spiritual health (in terms of "being at peace with oneself"). It is thus vital, in health promotion work, to take into account the subjective viewpoints of individuals (and communities) on health and to adopt a broad, holistic, model of health.

The state of health of a particular person, at any one point in time, is influenced by a huge range of factors, such as nutrition, housing, occupation, income, environment, relationships, education, access to health care and constitutional (heredity) factors. Thomas McKeown has demonstrated the very limited role that medicine has played in improving the health of populations (5). He emphasizes that for most diseases, prevention by control of their origins is cheaper, more humane and more effective than intervention by treatment after they occur. This in no way diminishes the importance of the medical function, for when people are ill they want all that is possible done for them. It does, however, mean that we must also invest in health promotion if we are to make further improvements in health in the future. (For a more detailed discussion on concepts and determinants of health, see the suggestions in the note at the end of this chapter (6).)

THE CONCEPT OF HEALTH GAIN AND INVESTING IN HEALTH PROMOTION

The UK government now has a strategy for improving the health of the population (7). This builds on the concept of "health gain". Dr Peter Brambleby has developed an extremely useful definition of health gain (8). He says that health gain is:

> A measurable improvement in health status, in an individual or population, attributable to earlier intervention.

For explanatory notes on this definition, see the note at the end of this chapter (9).

We must now invest in health gain for the future. Some areas for investment will be effective quite quickly—within the space of a few years. Other areas will take many years before the results show up, perhaps in the next generation and the next millennium. It is therefore crucial that we plan for the *right* investments. The areas for investment include diagnosis, treatment and health and social care, in addition to health promotion. So, for example, hip replacement operations (surgical treatment) and treatment of angina by drugs (drug treatment) may both result in health gains. Caring for vulnerable people in the community involves considering how best to enable them to live satisfying lives, and will bring health gains.

The main areas for investment in health promotion

Here we are concerned with identifying the main areas for investment in health promotion. They are:

1. The extension of services and policies which we know are effective; for example, in the preventive medical field we know that screening for raised blood pressure can detect people at risk of cardiovascular disease, and treatment is effective in reducing mortality. Measles vaccine is highly

effective, and this illness could be eradicated, in the same way as smallpox. To take another example, which is the joint responsibility of local and national government, good public transport would improve health by reducing the number of cars on the road, thus lessening pollution, reducing the stress of travelling for commuters and reducing road accidents. It could also reduce isolation for those who do not own cars and enable people to have access to affordable shopping and leisure facilities—all measures which improve health and well-being. There is good evidence from North America, Scandinavia and Japan that health promotion in the workplace can improve both the quality of working life for everyone and also improve productivity at the same time.

2. Improving standards of living—the greatest burden of ill-health falls on the poorest sections of the population. Reducing inequalities in living standards will both reduce inequalities in health and raise the overall health status of the population. All employers could re-examine their policies related to inequalities in pay.
3. Improving the environment—the quality of our air, water, beaches, and access to safe spaces for living at home and at work, for travel and leisure, are all areas for improvement.
4. Lifestyles—improving and spreading good practice on how to help people to modify their lifestyles; for example, reducing the numbers of people who smoke or are overweight, increasing levels of physical activity, and reducing alcohol and drug problems, are just a few examples of areas to be tackled. New approaches to helping people to change their health behaviours and lifestyles are enabling us to become more effective in this field.

It is important to note that investment is required in *all* these areas. The evidence suggests that they are mutually reinforcing: investing in one area results in bigger gains not only in that area but in the other areas too. So, for example, it is easier for people to take physical exercise when they are provided with environments which encourage them to do this—safe cycleways, safe play areas for children, unpolluted and attractive environments in which to play healthy games, or just walk and relax.

Why invest in health promotion?

Every organization will have its own reasons for investing in health promotion work, such as the following:

- Leisure services managers are interested in extending the use of their facilities to new groups of people through capturing the "health market".

- Social services professions are interested in removing barriers to access to recreational facilities (through, for example, the provision of affordable transport to facilities) for their clients.
- Medical staff and nurses are interested in improving the rehabilitation of patients who have had heart surgery, or in preventing health problems, such as osteoporosis in older women.
- Community outreach project workers are concerned with meeting the needs for health education and health information of some of the most vulnerable members of society.
- Managers and health professionals in NHS trusts are interested in fulfilling their contractual obligations for health promotion and could also be interested in extending their activities into new areas and competing for new health promotion contracts.
- Managers and occupational health staff in workplaces are interested in reducing sickness, absenteeism and accidents, in improving the motivation and performance of staff, and in encouraging the active participation of staff in workplace health policies and standards.
- Managers and workers in voluntary organizations are interested in maintaining and extending services for their clients and need to know how to penetrate the health market and how to advocate for the interests of their clients.
- Managers, teachers and governors in schools are interested in working in partnership with health service staff, the police, parents, voluntary organizations and community groups in order to improve health education and school policies related to the health and well-being of pupils and their staff.
- Commissioning managers are interested in finding better ways of involving local people in defining and meeting health promotion needs, in investing in new areas of effective health promotion and in improving the monitoring, evaluation and audit of health promotion activities in order to justify investments.

MANAGING FOR HEALTH GAIN

At the heart of managing for health gain is the health gain cycle, or spiral (since, hopefully, as health gains are made an uplifting spiral will be created and the starting point each time will be at a point where health has improved). This spiral is the management tool for controlling health gain. It is illustrated in Figure 1.1 and involves five major stages:

Stage 1 Needs assessment. (What are the areas for investment in health promotion, treatment, care and rehabilitation in order to make health gains? How can the needs best be met?)

Stage 2 Planning (What do we want to achieve? How are we going to achieve it? How will we know if we are succeeding?)
Stage 3 Implementation ("doing" the planned work).
Stage 4 Evaluation (showing whether we are on track, measuring the health gain).
Stage 5 Review. (How could we improve? What do we do next?)

This cycle or spiral may look "scientific", but it actually involves making a number of value judgements, because it means juggling competing pressures and constraints on what is actually possible in practice. So, for example, the public, different professions, and local and national politicians may all have different views about needs, priorities and how to improve practice. In addition, it is not possible for commissioners and purchasers to make huge shifts in the sort of activities they fund overnight. Hospitals cannot be closed down quickly; and developing effective preventive and health promotion measures may involve considerable research and development work to get it right. Last, but not least, in order to improve health we need to know about what it is that makes people healthy, since this may not be the same as what makes them sick. On the whole, we know a lot about the latter, but we don't know so much about what makes people have top-quality health and well-being (and therefore, how best to promote it).

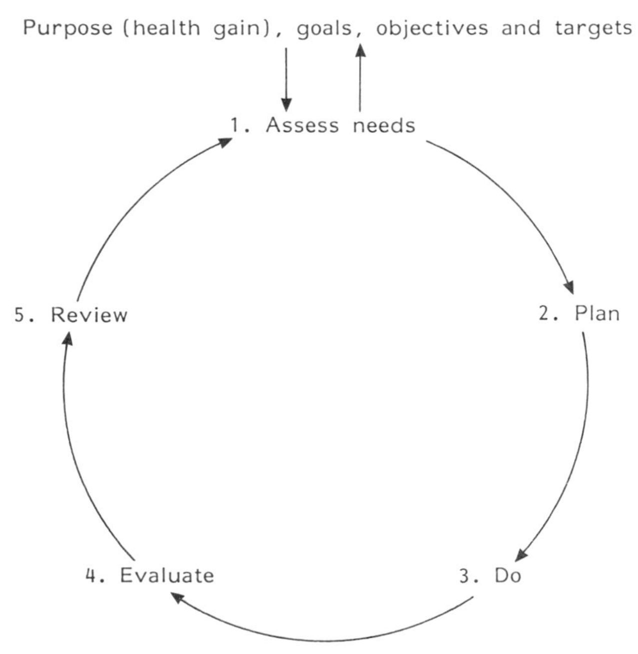

Figure 1.1 The health gain spiral

Financial profit or loss is the yardstick to assess a company's progress in the commercial world. Health gain is the equivalent for all the organizations playing a part in the national health strategy—the fundamental tool of management which measures our achievement of our common purpose. In Chapter 3 I discuss needs assessment, and in Chapter 6 I discuss in detail how to set goals, objectives and targets and how to evaluate health promotion activities.

THE MEANING OF HEALTH PROMOTION MANAGEMENT

The management of health promotion work thus involves achieving health gain through specific health promotion interventions, as opposed to other measures. The management of health promotion starts with the government and involves efforts by a range of agents at both national and local levels. The government, for example, has set up a joint Nutrition Task Force, which is a partnership of officials from relevant government departments and representatives from other sectors with an interest in food and nutrition. It is charged with harnessing and facilitating the contributions of all the agents and agencies concerned (see the following box).

Agents and opportunities for promoting healthy eating (Source: adapted from HM Government White Paper 1992) (10)

Agent/ agency	*Opportunity identified*
Health education authority	• Continuing to develop nutrition education resources.
Food producers, retailers	• Increasing the variety and availability of foods with low fat and sodium content. • Offering plentiful and easily accessible supplies of starchy staples, vegetables and fruit. • Introducing full nutrition labelling. • Developing marketing practices conducive to healthy food choices.
Caterers	• Offering menus which encourage people to choose healthy diets. • Using government nutritional guidelines. • Ensuring nutrition education and training of catering staff.

continued on next page

continued

Health/local authorities	• Ensuring health and dietetic expertise for the health, social services and education sectors. • Maximizing opportunities for educating people about healthy eating. • Using government nutritional guidelines in catering facilities.
Media/advertisers	• Giving the public information about healthy eating.
Voluntary sector	• Taking initiatives to encourage healthy eating. • Coordinating activities with others.

In this book I am primarily concerned with the management of health promotion work at local level but, of course, that involves taking account of what is going on at national level and in the wider environment.

It is not easy to define what *management* is, but in general terms we can say it is about being efficient and effective in health promotion work. *Effectiveness* is the extent to which the results you set out to achieve are actually achieved. *Efficiency* is about how you achieve those results compared with other ways of achieving them, for example whether the same results could be achieved more cheaply by doing things another way. Managing involves activities such as forecasting, planning, organizing, coordinating and controlling. Managerial activities are not confined to managers, because all work, whatever your profession or discipline, requires undertaking activities such as setting priorities, making sound decisions, planning, organizing, using information systems and controlling things such as use of resources. So managerial competencies are needed by everyone—in fact one could argue that they are a prerequisite for living! Managers are people who "specialize" in these managerial activities and get things done through other people, for example through front-line workers (such as the health and welfare professions). Often managers will retain some of their "doing" functions, as an expert or a professional, and thus have to manage the tension between the different parts of their job.

This book aims to improve the *management* of health promotion. It is thus aimed at more than just managers—it is aimed at all those people who have significant management responsibilities in their jobs, and therefore need to ensure "healthy" ways of working for themselves and their staff, and who actually, or potentially, are responsible for managing health promotion work and/or for allocating resources to health promotion. This includes business executives, general managers, and senior professionals and workers in a very wide range of professions and occupations. It is not, however, intended as a substitute for comprehensive management development and training, but seeks to raise awareness of the competencies required for meeting the challenges of health promotion. (For suggestions related to sources of management education and training, see the note at the end of this chapter (11).)

WORKING TOGETHER IN HEALTH-PROMOTING ORGANIZATIONS

There are two other fundamental aspects of managing health promotion which you will need to consider, if you are to be successful.

Working together for better health

Many of the activities we need to invest in for health gain through health promotion work can only be delivered through partnerships between organizations, and between organizations and communities, at local level. Liaison and cooperation between staff working for different agencies is obviously not new and happens in a myriad of different ways. Such "inter-agency working" includes all the ways in which organizations can work together. The term "health alliances" (health partnerships) means something more specific. I suggest a working definition below:

> Health alliances are two or more agencies working together to achieve health gain, which the agencies working on their own could not achieve as effectively or efficiently.

The purpose of any health alliance is thus to make a significant contribution to the achievement of health gain for local populations. This is done by building effective partnerships involving all the main agencies who have a role to play in particular aspects of health gain (such as the promotion of physical activity or the prevention of accidents). Some alliances will have a wholly health promotion focus; others will span across health promotion into other areas of health gain, such as diagnosing, treating or caring for people with particular health problems. I illustrate this through the example in the following box.

Example of a health alliance: Alcohol partnerships

Many partnerships on alcohol operate at local level in the UK and involve joint working by a range of agencies such as the police, the courts, brewers, licensees, the youth service, the probation service, social services, schools, voluntary organizations, local employers, occupational health staff, prison officers, consultant psychiatrists, NHS accident and emergency department staff, physicians, specialist health promotion staff, and others! Each of these agents and agencies will have their own unique objectives and areas of expertise (for example, a psychiatrist will have expertise on dependency and problem drinking). In order to work together, they need to identify *shared objectives*, many of which will focus on prevention/health promotion.

For example, research on reducing the harm from alcohol consumption suggests that interventions by the police, youth workers, probation officers and publicans might be expected to reach the very large numbers of hazardous drinkers who are not reached by screening strategies directed at the early problem drinker (12). However, not all publicans, or police, are convinced about the importance of taking on a health promotion role ("I didn't join the police to be a social worker"). So there is much work to be done by alcohol alliances, both to find effective ways of collaborating and reaching shared goals, and to convince potential partners that it is worthwhile investing in prevention.

These health alliances are often complex, operating at different levels both within and between organizations:

- At the strategic level, alliances between health commissioning agencies, health service providers, other local agencies such as local government, voluntary organizations, and representatives of local people, decide on priorities and goals, and what programmes they intend to fund to contribute to the goals. (For an explanation of what is a "health commissioning agency" and a "provider", see the note at the end of this chapter (13).)
- Providers then need to develop business plans for the particular services for which they are responsible.
- At operational management level, mechanisms for joint management of programmes, projects and services may need to be agreed.
- Finally, there is the practitioner/user level (the "front line"), at which the day-to-day activities of delivering the health promotion service or project are carried out by health promoters possibly in partnership with local people.

The Department of Health has issued useful guidance on how to work in partnerships, with examples from the work of existing health alliances (14).

However, learning how best to work together is probably the biggest challenge facing the management of health promotion activities, and is a recurring theme throughout this book. Managers may have the skills to direct and control their own staff. Working in alliances requires the skills to influence those over whom you have no control, to develop a shared ownership of programmes and projects, to agree plans and share resources, and the willingness to share the glory (or the brick-bats).

Health-promoting organizations

To be successful we need organizations which aim to promote health *in* and *through* themselves; that is, organizations which improve health because of the intrinsic ways in which they set about their work, as well as through undertaking particular health promotion activities—organizations which are good at mutual empowerment, both at empowering their own staff, their customers, users, students or suppliers, other organizations they work in partnership with, and the communities they serve—organizations which focus the efforts of empowered people on improving the health of all concerned. Such organizations can be termed "health-promoting organizations". It is *management* that will be the driving force in creating these organizations, for it is management that couples vision to action. The key characteristics of health-promoting organizations are as follows:

- The organizations are powerful at development and creating change: they anticipate change, they innovate for health, they adapt, and they modify the environment to maintain their success in health promotion.
- The managers and staff do not exercise power over people, but share power with people in order to achieve shared health benefits. Organizations that are managed in this way provide a role model for other organizations and indeed for how health promotion can be carried out across the whole community.
- The organizations prioritize the health and well-being of all those people with whom they are concerned, including managers and employees, patients/customers/users/students, and those working for suppliers or partner organizations.
- The organizations contribute to the health and well-being of the communities they serve, through, for example, contributing to the long-term maintenance and improvement of the environment.
- The organizations are committed to sharing their experience with others and thus contributing to the spread of health-promoting organizations and communities.

A checklist of key points for moving towards a health-promoting organization (15)

	Traditional health education	*The health-promoting organization*
1.	Considers health education only related to the improved health of individual users or employees.	Takes a wider view including all aspects of the activities of the organization and its relationship with the community.
2.	Emphasizes health and safety and physical health to the exclusion of wider aspects.	Is based on a concept of health which includes the interaction of physical, mental and social aspects.
3.	Lacks a coherent, coordinated approach which takes account of the wide range of influences on health.	Recognizes the wide range of influences on health, and takes account of cultural, socio-economic and environmental factors.
4.	Takes limited account of psychological factors in relation to health behaviour.	Views the development of a positive self-image and individuals taking increasing control of their lives as central to the promotion of good health.
5.	Does not consider the health and well-being of all those groups of people associated with the organization.	Recognizes the importance of the health and well-being of all those people associated with the organization, e.g. managers, directors, employees, patients/customers/users, suppliers, relatives, visitors, students, colleagues, partners, teachers and governors.
6.	Fails to actively involve all the groups of people who are associated with the organization.	Considers the active participation of all the groups of people who are associated with the organization as central to health promotion.
7.	Views the role of the occupational health services as concerned solely with screening and disease prevention.	Takes a wider view of occupational health services, as including health education, counselling, the implementation of healthy policies and practices, environmental improvements and building health alliances with other agencies and with the community.

I provide some examples of health-promoting organizations we could learn from in Chapter 8.

Working together in health-promoting organizations is best understood if it is seen as a goal, as a process for achieving that goal, and as a philosophy setting out the way health promotion should be managed. It is about building the infrastructure we need to achieve health development.

LINKING THE HEALTH AND ENVIRONMENT AGENDAS

Health commissioners and local government are now beginning to work together with local communities on the shared agenda of enabling improvements to the well-being and quality of life of local people. For a current example of this, see the suggestion for further reading in the note at the end of this chapter (16). One important way in which shared objectives can be forged is through using Agenda 21 (the agreements on sustaining the environment forged by governments at the Earth Summit in Rio de Janiero in 1992). This can become an over-arching theme, linking health and environmental agendas.

- Agenda 21 proposes a comprehensive programme of action needed throughout the world to achieve a more sustainable pattern of development for the next century. (For detailed information on the UK response to Agenda 21, see *Sustainable Development: The UK Strategy* (17). For an explanation of what is meant by "sustainable development" see the note at the end of the chapter (18).)
- Local authorities are required to prepare and publish, by 1996, local agenda 21 strategies (so called "Green" plans) which are wide-ranging policy statements and action plans to ensure a sustainable environment. There is scope for health authorities to work with local authority planning departments over local "Green" plans.

Health has been embedded in the concept of sustainable development since its beginning (19). Until recently, however, public health medicine and health promotion specialists have often not been actively engaged in decision-making or policy-setting on sustainable development. *We need to shift the emphasis on the environment and health from protecting humans from environmental hazards, to protecting equally the environment from human hazards.*

"Sustainability" is about justice across the generations and the fate of our own grandchildren. Local councils are wrestling with how to make it a reality. So, for example, Glasgow launched a "regeneration alliance" in 1993, and this is trying to steer the city in a just and more sustainable direction—by developing a light railway system, bringing derelict land into use, improving the landscape, investing in skills and manufacturing industries, and making the place better for all classes (20).

Those involved in health promotion could make valuable contributions to the sustainable environment debate (21), through their understanding of important factors such as:

- An appreciation of the limitations of scientific data, and that decision-making involves value judgements and is an ethical matter.
- A broad, holistic, concept of health, particularly the role of political/economic equity in creating individual and population health.
- An appreciation of the limitations of "lifestyle" strategies (strategies based only on individual lifestyle change).
- An understanding of the concept of mutual empowerment, its relationship to personal and community health, and its implications for sustainable development, such as enabling people to take increased responsibility for the environment.

Both health promotion and sustainable development encourage the development in communities of skills in community organizing, policy advocacy, and other forms of participatory democracy that constitute the larger personal responsibility of citizenship. In the final chapter of this book I focus on how you could play a wider role in harnessing such community participation.

Questions you could ask yourself

1. Why are you (and your business) interested in investing in health promotion work? What are the main areas you could consider investing in?
2. Consider the checklist of key points for moving towards a health-promoting organization. Where do you put your organization in relation to each of the points (rate your organization on a continuum of 1: traditional, to 10: fully health promoting)? What steps could you take to move further in the direction of a health-promoting organization?
3. Does your organization work together with any other organizations for the purpose of achieving health gains? Which additional organizations could you work in partnership with, and at what levels will it be necessary to establish links?

NOTES, REFERENCES AND FURTHER READING

(1) The meaning and scope of health promotion, including a suggested framework for categorizing health promotion activities, are discussed in:

Ewles, L. and Simnett, I. (3rd edn, 1995) *Promoting Health: A Practical Guide*. London: Scutari Press. Ch. 2. Note 5 at the end of Ch. 2 lists some of the key papers and books on the meaning of health promotion.

For a useful book on the theory of health promotion, which traces its theoretical roots in disciplines such as psychology, sociology, education and epidemiology, and provides examples of the practical application of theory, see:

Bunton, R. and Macdonald, G. (eds) (1992) *Health Promotion: Disciplines and Diversity*. London: Routledge.

(2) I offer the following working definition of health promotion:

> An umbrella term for a wide range of activities which enhance positive health and prevent ill-health, including health education, preventive measures, healthy public policies, environmental measures and community and organizational health development.

The World Health Organization defines health promotion as:

> The process of enabling people to increase control over, and to improve, their health.

I offer the following working definition of *health education*:

> An essential facet of health promotion, which aims to ensure that people are well informed about health issues, have the ability to make choices about their health and lifestyles, and have the skills to carry out actions and behaviours to pursue those choices. It also aims to raise awareness of the need for policy changes within organizations, including governments, and for environmental changes conducive to health.

(3) Health promotion empowers people through supporting personal and social development by, for example, providing health information, education for health and enhancing life skills. In this way, it increases the options available to people to exercise more control over their own health and over their environment, and to make choices conducive to health. At the same time, it improves the quality of relationships, so that they are based on mutual respect and produce benefits for all the partners. It is based on the principle that people need to learn throughout life, to prepare themselves for all of its stages and to cope with stress and illness. People feel "disempowered" (a lack or loss of power) for a variety of reasons, and it is important in health promotion work to develop sensitivity and awareness of what these reasons might be.

(4) Doyal, L. and Gough, I. (1991) *A Theory of Human Need*. London: Macmillan.

(5) McKeown, T. (2nd edn 1986) *The Role of Medicine: Dream, Mirage or Nemesis*. Oxford: Blackwell.

(6) See:

Ewles. L. and Simnett, I. (3rd edn, 1995) *Promoting Health: A Practical Guide.* London: Scutari Press. Ch. 1.

(7) HM Government White Paper (1992) *The Health of the Nation: A Strategy for Health in England.* London: HMSO (Cm. 1986).

The corresponding documents for the other parts of the UK are:

Northern Ireland: Department of Health and Social Services (1991) *A Regional Strategy for the Northern Ireland Health and Personal Social Services 1992–1997.* Belfast: HMSO.

Scotland: Scottish Office (1992) *Scotland's Health: A Challenge to Us All.* Edinburgh: HMSO.

Wales: Welsh Office (1989) *Strategic Intent and Direction for the NHS in Wales.* Cardiff: Welsh Office NHS Directorate/Welsh Health Planning Forum.

For further information on the UK health strategies, see Chapter 6. For a more detailed discussion on the UK strategies, see:

Ewles, L. and Simnett, I. (3rd edn 1995) *Promoting Health: A Practical Guide.* London: Scutari Press. Ch. 6.

(8) See the *Managing Health Improvement Project* (MAHIP) open learning materials: *Needs Assessment for Health Improvement and Health Gain* includes a unit on "The Concept of Health Gain", which was written by Peter Brambleby, and provides this definition.

For further information about the availability of these materials, which were commissioned by the Health Education Authority and the NHS Training Division, contact Professional Development, Health Education Authority, Hamilton House, Mabledon Place, London WC1H 9TX. Telephone: 0171 3833833.

(9) These explanatory notes are based on a more extensive discussion in the unit on "The Concept of Health Gain" which forms part of the volume *Needs Assessment for Health Improvement and Health Gain* in the *Managing Health Improvement Project* (MAHIP) open learning materials. For information about the availability of these materials, see note (8) above.

Measurable health gain means that we must use, or devise, instruments which will verify that a change has occurred.

Improvement means any positive change, including changes in the quality of life as well as the length of life.

Health status is a portfolio term, encompassing a multitude of indicators of health.

Individual or population—managers are concerned with health gain in groups, communities or populations. This is the sum of shifts in individuals, which may be up or down in particular cases.

Attributable—proving that changes are the result of specific health promotion activities can be very difficult to do, because there are so many other influences on health. This means that we must gather information on both the short-term and long-term impact of activities, in order to make any kind of informed judgement.

An earlier intervention—interventions are not restricted to *health or social care* interventions. As I have already discussed, the provision, for example, of safe environments for pedestrians and cyclists, by the local authority highways department will have more impact on road accidents than health service accident and emergency departments.

(10) HM Government White Paper (1992) *The Health of the Nation*: A Strategy for Health in England. London: HMSO. p. 54.

For further information on the Nutrition Task Force and its plans, see:

Nutrition Task Force (1994) *Eat Well! An Action Plan from the Nutrition Task Force to Achieve the Health of the Nation Targets on Diet and Nutrition*. London: Department of Health.

Copies are available from BAPS, Health Publications Unit, DSS Distribution Centre, Heywood Stores, Manchester Road, Heywood, Lancs OL10 2PZ.

(11) For further information on management, see:

Handy, C.B. (3rd edn, 1985) *Understanding Organizations*. Harmondsworth: Penguin Business Library.

National Extension College and Lucas Open Learning (1988) *How to Work Effectively: The Secret of Success in your Job*. London: Thorsons Publishing Group.

Young, A. (1986) *The Manager's Handbook*. London: Sphere Books.

For practical help for nurses, see:

Schudin, V. and Shober. J. (1990) *Managing Yourself*. London: Macmillan Education, Essentials of Nursing Management Series.

For practical help for hospital doctors who are working as managers, see:

Sutherst, J. and Glascott, V. (1994) *The Doctor-Manager*. Edinburgh: Churchill Livingstone.

For practical help for general practitioners on the management of general practice, see:

Gilligan, C. and Lowe, R. (1994) *Marketing and General Practice*. Oxford: Radcliffe Medical Press.

For help with the management of voluntary organizations, see:

Handy, C. (1988) *Understanding Voluntary Organizations*. Harmondsworth: Penguin.

For a practical handbook aiming to help people working in the voluntary sector to improve their working effectiveness, see:

Holloway, C. and Otto, S. (1985) *Getting Organized*. London: Bedford Square Press.

For a handbook on managing designed for both voluntary organizations and community groups, see:

Merritt, T. and Adironack, S. (1989) *Just about managing*? London: London Voluntary Service Council.

The Open College have designed a series of courses called Working Effectively. The courses include: Managing Time, Managing Stress, Making Presentations, Moving into Management—a course for women, Interviewing, and Managing Change. For further information contact: The Open College, Third Floor, St James Buildings, Oxford Street, Manchester, M1 6FQ.

The Open University Business School provides a comprehensive distance learning course in management—The Effective Manager. For further details contact The Open University, Open Business School, Walton Hall, Milton Keynes MK7 6AG. Telephone 01908 274066.

The NHS Training Division (NHSTD) has commissioned a comprehensive open learning scheme for health service managers—the Management Education Scheme by Open Learning (MESOL). It comprises two programmes: Managing Health Services (MHS) for first line managers in the health service; and Health and Social Services Management (HSSM), for middle and senior managers in health and social services (including statutory, voluntary and private sectors). These are available through the Open University and locally through some health authorities and colleges. For further information on the availability of MESOL programmes contact The Open University (address above) or The Institute of Health Services Management, 39 Chalton Street, London NW1 1JD. Telephone 0171 388 2626 or the NHSTD (address below).

The NHS Training Division has also commissioned Health Pickup. This is a modular training programme to develop the non-clinical (managerial) skills of health service professionals including nurses, midwives, health visitors, dietitians, physiotherapists, occupational therapists, speech therapists, clinical psychologists and chiropodists. It includes modules on setting objectives and standards, assessing needs and priorities, managing caseload and time, and effective teamworking, plus modules on Information Management and Technology aimed at a wider range of health service staff. For further information on the availability of Health Pickup contact the NHSTD, St Bartholomews Court, 18 Christmas Street, Bristol BS1 5BT. Telephone 0117 9291029.

Management education and training are also widely available from institutions of higher education.

(12) The importance of inter-agency working is emphasized in a number of reports and books on preventing the harm from alcohol. See, for example:

Faculty of Public Health Medicine of the Royal College of Physicians (1991) *Alcohol and the Public Health*. London: Macmillan.

Department of Health (1989) *Interdepartmental Circular on Alcohol Misuse*. London: DHSS.

Robinson, D., Tether, P. and Teller, J. (1989) *Preventing Alcohol Problems: A Guide for Local Action*. London: Tavistock.

The Masham Report emphasizes the importance of collaboration related to alcohol consumption in young people and crime prevention:

Home Office (1987) *Young People and Alcohol: Report of the Working Group of the Standing Conference on Crime Prevention*. London: Home Office.

Research in the UK suggests that health promotion related to drinking can be effective when it is focused on changing the attitudes and actions of those people and organizations in a position to directly influence the behaviour of drinkers. See, for example:

Jeffs, B. and Saunders, W. (1983) Minimising alcohol-related offences by enforcement of the existing licensing legislation. *British Journal of Addiction* **78**: 67–77.

(13) A *commissioner* is any organization or individual with a responsibility to identify the needs of a geographically defined population and to determine ways in which these needs could be met within available resources.

Health commissioning is therefore the process by which the health needs of a population are defined and appropriate services purchased and evaluated, in order to ensure maximum health gain. The role of the district health authority was changed as a result of the health service reforms set out in the NHS and Community Care Act 1990. Health authorities now have a statutory role as health commissioners. In addition, local authorities act as health commissioners through enabling the development of services such as housing, pollution control, health and safety, food safety, planning and building control, transport, education and social services.

More recently, *joint commissioning* has begun to emerge. This could be by health authorities merging with Family Health Services Authorities (FHSAs) (statutory bodies responsible for planning and administering primary care services for a geographically defined population coterminous with metropolitan district and shire county boundaries), and with neighbouring health authorities, to form *health commissions* with joint organizational structures and more purchasing power in the health marketplace (formal merger cannot take place until new legislation is in place, and is expected in 1996).

Local authorities and health authorities/health commissions have in some cases developed wider joint commissioning arrangements for Care in the Community and Health Promotion.

The agencies which provide health services are often referred to as *"providers"*. NHS Trusts are bodies providing hospital and/or community services. They are self-governing bodies with their own Boards of Directors and they negotiate contracts with *"purchasers"* (commissioners). GP fundholders are both purchasers and providers, because they directly provide a range of health care services and also purchase some health services on behalf of their patients (rather than these services being purchased by the local health authority/commission). This means that GP fundholders can "shop around" to find the best services to meet patients' needs.

Many other agencies act as providers of health promotion work, in addition to health services, such as environmental health services, social services, contracted-out local authority leisure services, local workplaces, educational institutions, and voluntary organizations.

(14) Department of Health (1993) *Working Together for Better Health*. London: Department of Health.

(15) This checklist is adapted from a list of key points for school management in moving from traditional school health education towards the health-promoting school. The list first appeared in the Scottish Health Education Group/Scottish Consultative Council on the 1989 curriculum. It is reproduced in Whitehead, M. (1989) *Swimming Upstream: Trends and Prospects in Education for Health*. London: King's Fund Institute. p. 20.

(16) See, for example:

Middleton, J. and Pulford, M. (1994) Sick Building Syndrome. *Health Service Journal* **104** (5411): 30–31 (14 July 1994).

(17) HM Government White Paper (1994) *Sustainable Development: The UK Strategy*. London: HMSO. Cm. 2426.

(18) The World Commission on Environment and Development defines sustainable development as:

development that meets the needs of the present without compromising the ability of future generations to meet their own needs.

(19) World Commission on Environment and Development (1987) *Our Common Future*. Oxford: Oxford University Press.

(20) "Global justice begins at home". A report by David Donnison in *The Guardian*, Society pull-out, p. 3, November 23 1994.

(21) Labonté, R. (1991) Econology: Integrating Health and Sustainable Development. Part Two: Guiding Principles for Decision-making. *Health Promotion International* **6**(2): 147–156.

CHAPTER 2 How you can get from where you are to where you want to be

Summary

The chapter starts by examining some of the reasons why we need to develop health-promoting organizations. It introduces the concept of "value-adding management" and describes some performance indicators which can be used to assess how successful organizations are at becoming health-promoting. It then looks at how you can critically examine and evaluate your own approach to developing a health-promoting organization, through asking yourself some important questions. It moves on to discuss why changing bureaucratic structures into more flexible and adaptable ones is important for health-promoting organizations. It then discusses the process of health development and identifies some key factors related to the successful introduction of developments. Finally, it describes five stages in designing a strategy for implementing major developments: stage 1—joining together; stage 2—diagnosis; stage 3—vision: stage 4—developing ourselves; stage 5—setting an action plan. It emphasizes that a key element of the action plan will be a communication strategy, because without good communication any change will flounder. It ends with some questions you could ask yourself.

THE NEED FOR HEALTH DEVELOPMENT

As we have seen in Chapter 1, health promotion is about developing the potential of people to take increased responsibility for their own, and others', health. This means starting with developing the health potential of your own staff. Sir John Harvey-Jones, speaking at the NHS Training Division's annual convention in July 1994, stated that no organization he had visited in the UK thought that it was using more than 50% of its staff's capability (1). He contends that this has resulted in a great "poverty of aspiration" and that remedying this will require big changes in organizations in the UK whatever their business. Reorientating the NHS towards investing more resources in the promotion of better health, and to achieving more health benefits for people, rather than concentrating efforts just on the provision of health services, is one example of such a challenge. Meeting this challenge will require health development at a number of levels:

- *Personal health development*: the development of individual people's potential to take responsibility for their own, and others', health.
- *Professional health development*: establish sound principles on which health practitioners can base their health promotion practice, spread good practices and improve competence in health promotion work.
- *Organizational health development*: the development of health-promoting organizations.
- *Health development in and through alliances*: the development of health-promoting partnerships.
- Community health development: the development of health *in* and *through* communities ("health-promoting communities").

Bruce Tofield, in a recent article in *The Independent*, uses the concept of *value-adding management* (management which adds value to an organization, and to the people it employs and serves, through improving its performance) (2). He emphasizes that value-adding management does not come just through management training (although this has an important part to play) but is fundamentally related to the manner in which people develop the capacity to make good judgements and wise decisions in the face of complexity. One step towards creating more value-adding management is through identifying indicators of success which characterize its application. These indicators can be used to assess the performance of management in moving towards "health-promoting organizations" (I discussed the concept and characteristics of health-promoting organizations in Chapter 1). Tofield suggests the following four key indicators:

- *Employee satisfaction*: employees gain fulfilment from their work, which utilizes their creativity and gives a sense of achievement. (Initiatives by managers which could contribute to this include mechanisms for consultation with staff about moving towards becoming a health-promoting organization and staff participation in how the necessary developments are implemented.)
- *Stewardship of the environment*: the organization is concerned to sustain the environment in which it lives, because it thinks long term and appreciates that the environment influences health (for example, through policies which sustain the biodiversity of life in the land owned by the organization, and policies which reduce the pollution caused by the organization).

- *Absence of discrimination*: there is no discrimination, because it is inefficient and diminishes effectiveness, and fails to tap the full health potential of staff. (For example, discrimination against women can be reduced through initiatives such as job sharing and career breaks, and through initiatives which develop their potential as leaders of health-promoting organizations.)
- *Beneficial reciprocal long-term relationships between the organization and other organizations and key people*: such as relationships between purchasers and providers, providers and their suppliers, managers and their employees, providers and their customers or users, and between organizations and key groups in the local community. For example, printing for an organization is done by other local organizations employing disabled people; managers invest in a better deal for staff, through inviting suggestions from staff for interventions which will improve their health, well-being and quality of working life; an organization joins the local health alliance which is taking action towards a "healthy" city or a "healthy" town.

One example, which illustrates the simultaneous operation of two of these key indicators (stewardship of the environment and beneficial relationships with staff and service users), has been taken by the Brighton Health Promotion Service, which has built a garden for use by staff and visitors. This helps to sustain biodiversity and at the same time promotes the mental health of users, through providing an environment in which they can relax and refresh themselves.

Any organization can use these four indicators to do a quick non-financial "health check" on its performance.

ASSESSING YOUR APPROACH TO DEVELOPING HEALTH-PROMOTING ORGANIZATIONS

How you approach the process of developing a health-promoting organization will be an important performance indicator. Your "mental model" of the development process will influence whether you are effectively able to achieve concrete and specific goals within the practical constraints and opportunities of your situation (3). Obviously, your model will be based to some extent on theory. Unfortunately, there is often a gulf between theory and practice which requires bridging. So, for example, a good theoretical analysis does not necessarily lead to a good design of a health development programme.

One way of raising your awareness of how you approach health development is through examining the logical structure of your arguments.

This can help to interpret and uncover the assumptions you make (4). You start by questioning the breadth and depth of your diagnosis, and the nature of the evidence, assumptions and conclusions which you have used. Next you look at the links between the diagnosis, the proposed development strategy, and the expected outcomes. Questions using this method, which will enable you to critically examine how you approach health development, are set out in the following box (5).

Examples of questions to ask yourself when evaluating your approach to developing a health-promoting organization

1. Adequacy of diagnosis
   - Have you adequately defined the need for developing a health-promoting organization?
   - Have you obtained appropriate and sufficient evidence to evaluate the nature of the health development needs?
   - Have you drawn reasonable conclusions from the evidence?
2. Value of expected outcomes
   - Are the expected outcomes realistically attainable?
   - Are the expected outcomes worth pursuing?
   - Do the expected outcomes appeal to any of the people with an interest? (For example, will the outcomes appeal to your staff or to your health commissioner?)
3. Appropriateness of health development strategy
   - Have you considered alternative strategies?
   - Does the selected strategy seem appropriate?
   - Is the selected strategy practical?
4. Compatibility of diagnosis, health development strategy and expected outcomes
   - Is the strategy compatible with the diagnosis?
   - Do the expected outcomes specifically result from the strategy?

ORGANIZATIONAL STRUCTURES AND HEALTH DEVELOPMENT

Since the 1960s many of the dominant theoreticians have focused their attention on factors relating to the *structure* of organizations, rather than on *processes*. Organizational structure includes factors such as the allocation of work, levels in the organizational hierarchy, and lines of communication and control (6). In an effective organization these factors reflect and reinforce the organization's goals and objectives. The results of some of the key research findings are set out in the following box.

Key research findings on organizational structures

- One study contrasted rigid bureaucratic structures with flexible matrix structures, and suggested that the former is typical of organizations characterized by stability and continuity with the past, and the latter is typical of innovative organizations (7). In a bureaucracy the emphasis on rules and procedures means that members are more concerned with the means of working than the ends or outcomes of their efforts.
- Another study placed the firms they studied along a continuum of very bureaucratic to very "organic" (flexible and adaptable) and concluded that "organic" firms were more suited to change and development (8). They found that "organic" firms are characterized by factors such as the following:
  - Tasks stem from the whole job to be done and are defined through team working.
  - Staff are not given a limited field of responsibility (for example, through job descriptions).
  - Communication consists of information and guidance, rather than instructions or decisions.
  - Shared decision-making.
  - High participation and interaction.
  - Many ideas are generated from the "bottom up".
  - Open communication laterally and up and down.

"Organic" structures are thus the ones most appropriate for health-promoting organizations. For example, as I have already pointed out, the NHS has in the past been more concerned with outputs (the provision of health services) than with outcomes (the improved health of the population it serves). Developing the NHS to achieve greater health benefits will require that the organizations constituting it are innovative and can realize the potential of their human resources. Developing public sector organizations, and other organizations, from bureaucracies into more flexible and adaptable organizations is thus a key aspect of health development, necessary for the successful implementation of health gain strategies.

We have already seen some welcome developments in this direction. For example, professions such as nursing have witnessed an expanding field of responsibility, such as nurse prescribing, and a reduction of autocracy. Outside the NHS, successful companies are currently breaking down bureaucracies and hierarchies, and examples are provided in the following box.

Examples of commercial companies with "organic" structures

- The new Xerox company uses informal cross-boundary and non-hierarchical groups to do everything from solving current problems to generating corporate policy, rather than relying on an organizational hierarchy.
- The new General Electric is more concerned with "liberating" people than with performance-related pay.

The recent results of both these companies show the benefits both in terms of the performance of the companies (profits) and in terms of improved well-being and quality of working life for their staff.

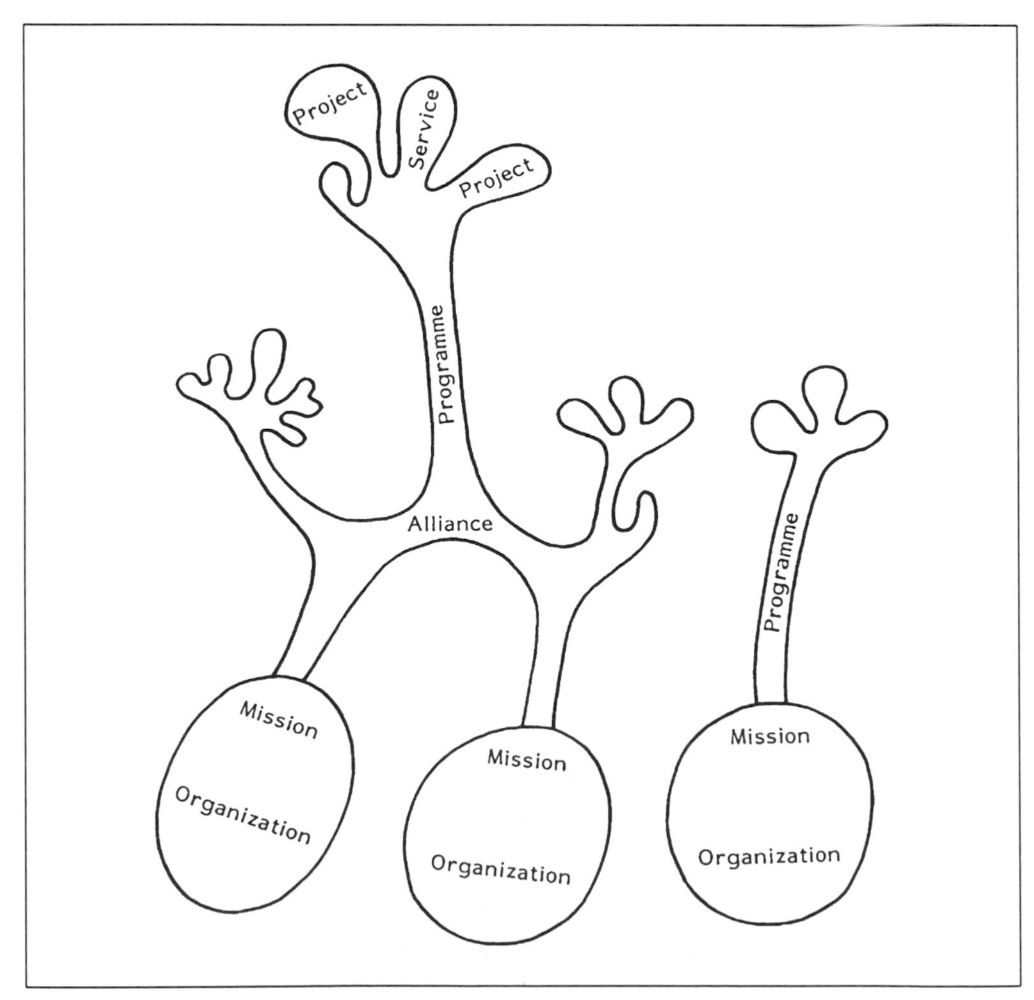

Figure 2.1 "Organic" development

So, the organizational hierarchies, which have been such a feature of the public sector, are being cast aside. Led by people like Dian-Marie Hosking (9) of Aston University and Helen Brown (10) of the Office for Public Management, and in North America by Robert Eccles (11), they are being replaced by a "new management" approach based on collaboration and a win–win philosophy. (The competencies required to "operationalize" this are explored in Chapter 7.) Arguably, top-down hierarchical management is inconsistent with public service professionalism, and with flexible and responsive service provision and active participation by citizens (12).

"Organic" development is illustrated in Figure 2.1.

THE PROCESS OF HEALTH DEVELOPMENT (13)

Development in organizations is often initiated by individuals or groups who have become aware of a mismatch between the demands of a changing environment and the current performance of the organization. If health developments are to be successfully implemented then the need for development must gain legitimacy. Agents of development using "new management" approaches do not, however, try to force through developments against the desires of the other interest groups; rather they develop the skills to intervene in the political and cultural systems of the organization concerned in order to build up a nucleus of political support.

The proponents of "new management" see development not as the outcome of power struggles between interest groups, but as a consequence of networking by managers and professionals inside and outside their organizations, in order to build clarity about what is important, and to support each other in working out what is going on and what to do about it. The advocates of new management thus stress power sharing. This philosophy is in line with the concept of health-promoting organizations which I have been developing. In addition, organizations with these characteristics will be more successful in establishing the collaborative partnerships and alliances which are essential, as I explained in Chapter 1, if we are to achieve health gains. "New management" thinking emphasizes that organizations which operate successfully in this way are likely to have three binding forces and we can therefore take these as key factors for creating health-promoting organizations. They are set out in the following box.

The key factors for creating a health-promoting organization

- Clarity about the overall purpose of the organization.
- A widely shared vision of a better future.
- A set of values and principles which govern the way it operates

The following sections of this chapter describe how to set about health development in such a way that these key criteria will be met.

Key factors for successful development

The key to gaining commitment to change, and overcoming resistance to new developments, lies in understanding the motivation of all the people who could be affected and how they feel about it. Overall, do they feel positive or negative about the proposed developments? The balance between positive and negative factors can be expressed as follows, in a "change equation" developed as a pseudo-mathematical tool to help analyse the key factors involved (14).

A = the individual's or group's level of dissatisfaction with things as they are now;
B = the individual's or group's shared vision of a better future;
C = the existence of an acceptable, safe first step;
D = the perceived costs to the individual or group.

Change is likely to be viewed positively, and be implemented successfully, if:

$$A + B + C \text{ is greater than } D$$

The basis of the equation is the simple assumption that people are rarely interested in change unless the factors supporting change outweigh the costs. As a change agent your job is either to reduce D, the perceived costs, or to increase the sum of A, B and C. For a more detailed discussion of the use of this technique, in the context of health promotion, see the reference at the end of the chapter (15).

DESIGNING A HEALTH DEVELOPMENT STRATEGY

The literature on the management of development and change is vast, and I make some suggestions about further reading at the end of this chapter (16). Here, I move on to describe some of the important stages in designing a health development strategy (i.e., a strategy for major developments towards a health-promoting organization, or a health-promoting partnership, or a health-promoting community).

This could be used to develop a strategy to manage developments, such as:

- Expanding your field of health promotion work.
- Changing your status to become an independent health promotion agency (rather than remaining as part of your existing organization).

- Playing an active part in improving the health of the local community.
- Making major changes in your staffing levels, such as directly employing only the staff responsible for "core" functions and contracting out non-core work.
- Introducing continuous quality management of all your health promotion activities.
- Changing your organizational structure to a more health-promoting one (a flatter one) and developing staff to work in autonomous teams.
- Developing partnerships and ways of joint working with other agencies and/or with local people and the community focused on health gain.
- Creating a learning organization focused on improved health and well-being and quality of working life.
- Improving the health of your staff, through finding out what developments in the workplace would be conducive to their improved health, and working together to implement them.

Stage 1: Join with others—identify the group who will manage the health development

Health development will require the commitment of a "management group". The importance of involving all the managers who will be concerned with health development right from the start cannot be over-emphasized. Ensuring the early involvement of all these managers is the first stage in gaining their commitment. However, they will all start from different positions, and this needs to be borne in mind. Commitment develops through the interaction of all the group members, not from pressure by the leader or chairperson, and will only grow if the group develops successfully. It will therefore be vital for the group leader to have good skills in group processes (17).

Stage 2: Diagnosis—where are we now and what changes do we forecast?

It is also vital to avoid the temptation to be too "solution-centred". The early stages of introducing strategic health developments involve reflection and cannot be skipped. The second stage involves the management group in reflecting on issues such as:

- How are things now—what are we satisfied with, and what are we dissatisfied with?

- How would we like things to be different?
- What external factors (outside our organization) are likely to change in the near future?
- What internal factors (inside our organization) are likely to change in the near future?
- What are the gaps in our forecast and how could we fill them?

All organizations are affected by external changes—social, technological, economic and political (STEP factors). Well-run organizations are constantly on the look-out for these STEP factors, and have a good intelligence network to keep them up to date. They forecast the likely impact of these factors on their activities, and adjust their activities when necessary—this is the process of strategic management. It starts with strategic *thinking* and it is the quality of this thinking which is crucial for developing a successful strategy.

Stage 3: Vision—where do we want to go?

The next stage is also a thinking phase, but it is essential to separate it, at this point in time, from the previous stage, so that the group does not act like a victim of the changes in its circumstances which it predicts, but creates a vision of where it would really like to be, based on its values, principles and views about the purpose of the organization. One way of handling this is actually to *reverse* stages 2 and 3, and to start by looking at where you want to be. Whether or not you do that, what you *must* do is to invent the future—"This is how we intend things to be." With good foresight and careful planning, plus the flexibility to assimilate unexpected events and to see challenges as opportunities, you really can create what you want! Effective development managers are people who are not overwhelmed by external forces, but can see them as starting points for growth and development. (See the case study of "*Healthy Oxford 2000*" in Chapter 8, for a personal account of how this happened.)

Your vision could include:

- Becoming an organization that promotes health as part of the way it works, as well as a place where health promotion activities take place.
- Less stress and anxiety amongst staff, users/patients (or students in educational institutions) and visitors.
- Reduced accidents and sickness, reduced staff turnover, increased job satisfaction, improved morale.
- An innovative workforce, capable of meeting new health challenges.
- Improved links with the local community, and an improved reputation.

- Improved and demonstrable quality of health promotion work.
- Improved impact on the health of the population or people you serve.
- More efficient use of local resources for health gain through working together with other local organizations.

Stage 4: Developing ourselves—how do we need to develop to make sure we get there?

Development is difficult because no one is a perfectly empowered person, and we all have things we need to learn. So, it is vital for the management group to identify both individual and shared development needs, and how help could be obtained in meeting these needs. The group members themselves will have many strengths and resources which they can share with each other, but it is likely that sometimes bringing in an external consultant, or buying in training, may be required. Perhaps the most important thing is developing the level of trust within the group itself so that group members can support each other. Coping with change and development at an emotional level can be the most difficult part. Developing oneself is often painful (I speak from very painful experience!) and support can therefore be crucial.

Stage 5: Action plan—how could we get there?

This stage involves setting an action plan. One key element of the plan should be to design a *communication* strategy, because communication is the life-blood of development, and without it any other plans are likely to flounder.

At a health development strategy level good communication has a vital contribution to make to a number of key functions:

- *Controlling*—ensuring that people work in a coordinated way towards a common goal.
- *Informing*—ensuring that people know what is going on and what is expected of them.
- *Integrating*—unifying everyone in a shared vision of a better future and maintaining morale.
- *Innovating*—ensuring the spread of ideas throughout the organization so that it can create, adapt and survive.

All of these functions are necessary during strategic health developments, so your communication strategy needs to tap into the right ones at the right time.

Another element of your action plan will be *target setting*. When designing your strategy, you need to set realistic, achievable targets, and identify stepping-stones towards the targets, based on your analysis of the helping and hindering forces, using techniques such as the "change equation". (Target setting is discussed further in Chapter 6.)

You may wish to undertake one or more *pilot projects*. In pilot projects, specific changes are made for a fixed period of time on an experimental basis. The effects of the change are then analysed using "before" and "after" criteria, to assess the outcome of the change. This is also a way of testing whether the proposed change is feasible and acceptable to all those concerned. Pilot changes require close supervision and monitoring, and should therefore be small scale, in order to ensure that this level of supervision can be maintained by the managers.

Finally, you must make detailed plans for each *stepping stone*, including plans for monitoring and reviewing progress on a regular basis, so that you can ensure that you keep on course. I look in more detail at what some of these stepping-stones might be in the next chapter. (The principles of planning and evaluation are discussed in more detail in Chapter 6.)

It is important to note that it may be necessary regularly to revisit these five stages of strategic health development, because some of the changes may take years and, for example, the management group may need to change its membership, or to renew its commitment to developing a health-promoting organization, or health-promoting partnerships, or a health-promoting community, and to improve the vision of what this means.

Questions you could ask yourself

1. How do you rate the performance of your organization as a "health-promoting organization" on the four key performance indicators suggested by Tofield (employee satisfaction, stewardship of the environment, absence of discrimination, and beneficial long-term reciprocal relationships with key organizations and people)? Can you think of anything you could do to improve performance related to these indicators?
2. Think of one health promotion development which you recently introduced in your organization. How do you rate yourself on:
   - Your diagnosis of the need for health development?
   - The value of the expected health outcomes?
   - The appropriateness of the health development strategy?
   - The compatibility of the diagnosis, the expected health outcomes and the health development strategy?

   How could you improve your strategic thinking?

continued on next page

continued

3. How do you rate the current performance of your organization in communicating on aspects of health promotion related to each of the strategic functions: controlling, informing, integrating and innovating? What could be done to improve communication?
4. Make some notes about the following:
   - What is the purpose of the organization I work for?
   - What is my vision of the organization as a health-promoting one?
   - Who shares this vision?
   - What values and principles which govern the way the organization operates could make a contribution to moving towards a health-promoting organization?

NOTES, REFERENCES AND FURTHER READING

(1) Quoted in the editorial in the *Health Service Journal* **104** (5413): 17 (28 July 1994).

(2) Tofield, B. The crucial hunt for tomorrow's company. *The Independent*, 15 March 1994, p. 30.

(3) Egan, G. (1985) *Change Agent Skills in Helping and Human Service Settings*. Monterey, CA: Brooks/Cole.

(4) Toulmin, S. (1958) *The Uses of Argument*. Cambridge: Cambridge University Press.

(5) These questions are adapted from questions in:

Spurgeon, P. and Barwell. F. (1991) *Implementing Change in the NHS*. London: Chapman & Hall, in association with the Health Services Management Centre.

(6) Hierarchies are a way of organizing which involves distributing authority in an ascending series of grades or levels, the top level retaining the most authority and discretion. A typical organizational hierarchy will be pyramid-shaped, with a few powerful individuals at the top but many individuals, each possessing little authority, in the lowest grades.

(7) Nystrom, H. (1979) *Creativity and Innovation*. Chichester: Wiley.

(8) Burns, T. and Stalker, G.M. (3rd edn, 1994) *The Management of Innovation*. Oxford: Oxford University Press.

(9) Hosking, D. M. (1992) *A Social Psychology of Organising*. London: Harvester.

(10) Brown, H. (1992) *Women Organising*. London: Routledge.

(11) Eccles, R. (1992) *Beyond the Hype*. Harvard: Harvard Business School.

(12) For an overview of the impact of managerialism on public services, including case studies, see:

Farnham, D. and Horton, S. (eds) (1993) *Managing the New Public Services*. Basingstoke: Macmillan.

(13) This section is based on material and ideas which I develop in more depth in *Management Competencies for Health Gain*, which is part of the *Managing Health Improvement Project* (MAHIP) open learning material. For information about the availability of these materials, see note (8) in Chapter 1.

In addition, some of the information is adapted from study texts forming part of the *Certificate in Health Education Open Learning Resources*, London: Health Education Authority 1993.

(14) Open Business School (1990) *Managing Health Services*. Milton Keynes: The Open University. Book 9: *Managing Change*, pp. 36–37.

(15) Ewles, L. and Simnett, I. (3rd edn, 1995) *Promoting Health: A Practical Guide*. London: Scutari Press. Ch. 7.

(16) The following suggestions are recent publications, which provide an introduction to the field.

Drennan, D. (1992) *Transforming Company Culture: Getting your Company from Where you Are Now to Where you Want to Be*. London: McGraw-Hill.

Drucker, P.F. (1992) *Managing for the Future*. Oxford: Butterworth-Heinemann.

Handy, C. (2nd edn, 1991) *The Age of Unreason*. London: Century Business.

Handy, C. (1994) *The Empty Raincoat: Making Sense of the Future*. London: Hutchinson.

Kanter, R.M. (1989) *When Giants Learn to Dance: Mastering the Challenge of Strategy, Management and Careers in the 1990s*. London: Simon & Schuster.

Kanter, R.M., Stein, B.A. and Todd, D.J. (1992) *The Challenge of Organization Change: How Companies Experience it and Leaders Guide it*. New York: Free Press.

Morgan, G. (1988) *Riding the Waves of Change: Developing Managerial Competencies for a Turbulent World*. San Francisco: Jossey-Bass.

Pascale, R. (1991) *Managing on the Edge*. Harmondsworth: Penguin.

Peters, T. (1989) *Thriving on Chaos*. London: Macmillan.

Peters, T. (1993) *Liberation Management: Necessary Disorganization for the Nanosecond Nineties*. London: Pan Books, in association with Macmillan.

Stewart, R. (1991) *Managing Today and Tomorrow*. London: Macmillan.

(17) For an introduction to working with groups and suggestions for further reading, see:

Ewles, L. and Simnett, I. (3rd edn, 1995) *Promoting Health: A Practical Guide*. London: Scutari Press. Ch. 9

See also the section on "*How to build health-promoting teams*" in Chapter 7.

CHAPTER 3 The stepping-stones of health development

Summary

This chapter looks at some of the key stepping-stones towards creating "health-promoting organizations" and healthy partnerships. It starts by discussing how you can improve your own health development potential, through enhancing your abilities to be flexible and adaptable and to empower others, and through improving your managerial and personal health development skills. It then discusses how to move towards a more flexible organizational design, through using three key principles: strengthening of teamworking, semi-autonomous teams, and reducing the management structure above team level. It continues by highlighting that this will mean prioritizing staff training and development. It discusses the meaning of competence and explains the benefits a competence-based approach to staff assessment and development will bring. It moves on to explain how you could analyse the health promotion role of your staff, through undertaking a role-mapping exercise, and use this to improve their work performance. It then describes a number of key issues which commissioners must consider when formulating health gain strategies. The final sections describe how providers could become involved in a health promotion strategy, through working in their own setting and through working in health partnerships. It ends with an activity you could undertake, related to the development of teams, and some questions you could ask yourself related to your own development.

IMPROVING YOUR OWN HEALTH DEVELOPMENT POTENTIAL

We have already seen, in Chapter 2, that moving towards health-promoting organizations and effective health alliances is a big job. The best place to start is probably with yourself. The better at "health-promoting" management you can become, the more effective you will be as a role model for others. You could start by reflecting on your approach to management and how it could be improved in order to bring health benefits for yourself and others. The way you behave will be based on the views of the world you have built up as a result of your experiences. By recognizing the factors which have influenced you in the past, you can "reframe" reality, break the links with past experiences, and choose more freely how you will behave in future. In other words, you can empower yourself to take more responsibility for choosing how to behave in different situations, and thus become more flexible and adaptable.

One way of increasing your awareness of your management behaviour is to work out how strongly you are influenced by different factors. These include personal characteristics, such as how far you believe yourself to be in control or how far you see yourself as controlled by your organization, or by other people. The more you believe yourself to be controlled externally (by events, fate, other people or circumstances) the more this will be a self-fulfilling prophecy. How valuable do you consider yourself to be? A low sense of self-esteem not only means that you could be over-critical of yourself, and under-estimate your own abilities, but you could also under-estimate the abilities of your staff and other people.

Another set of influences on your approach to management will be the habitual ways you have built up in dealing with other people. McGregor has described two basic approaches to dealing with other people, which he refers to as theory X and theory Y.(1) Managers or professionals operating on theory X believe other people to be lazy, resistant to change and in need of being pushed around. Managers or professionals operating from theory Y believe that people have the potential to develop and change and are motivated by being given responsibility and by the satisfaction of "a job well done". Theory Y managers/professionals see their role as an enabling one—providing the conditions in which staff or colleagues can best direct their own efforts towards agreed (in our case, health) goals and objectives. Theory Y managers/professionals thus seek to empower others and in so doing contribute towards the improved health and well-being of others.

The ability to empower others, while remaining empowered yourself, is closely linked to assertiveness. Assertiveness is about gaining win–win situations through direct and open communication and through avoiding aggressive behaviour (win–lose situations) or manipulation (lose–lose situations). It builds the sense of self-esteem of all concerned. For further reading on how to develop your assertiveness, and on how to develop yourself, see the suggestions at the end of the chapter (2).

Some of the personal development skills ("life skills") required to enable you to improve your own, and others', health and well-being are discussed in the section on "Developing life skills" in Chapter 9.

You may also wish to improve particular managerial skills necessary for health development. For example, you may wish to improve your skills in handling meetings, which take up so much time. The pressures of, and ineffectiveness of, many meetings are requiring managers and professionals to move away from regular, calendar-driven meetings, towards issue-driven meetings, which are only held when they are really necessary. Or you may wish to improve your ability to produce good written documents, such as position papers, business plans and reports; or to improve your use of information technology. Suggestions on sources of help related to these, and other, managerial skills are provided in the note at the end of the Chapter (3). Some of the key managerial skills and abilities required for health development are discussed in Chapter 7.

For further reading on how to develop your management abilities, directly through your own managerial experiences, see the suggestions in the note at the end of the chapter (4).

DEVELOPING HEALTH-PROMOTING ORGANIZATIONS

I have already discussed, in Chapter 2, how changing the design of an organization can play a part in improving the way the work is managed and can at the same time contribute towards health gain for all concerned. Any organization needs to carry out a number of key functions:

1. *Strategic planning*: high-level scanning activity, such as looking at major factors likely to impact on health and health promotion, and deciding how these issues should be addressed in strategy and policy-making (5). Much of the intelligence on these factors can be gathered "from the bottom up" within the organization, but good intelligence networks are also essential for identifying wider influences.
2. *Business planning*: a plan which is market-orientated and service-driven, produced by analysing where the business is now, where it is going, whether it has the ability to get there, how it is going to do it, how much it will cost and whether it is worthwhile. An important feature of the plan will be the clear identification of key results (programme) areas for health promotion work.
3. *Operational management*: a system for organizing the delivery of health promotion programmes, ensuring clarity about where the lead lies for each programme area and clarity about roles and responsibilities.
4. *Quality improvement*: a system for ensuring that key results are achieved without waste and duplication of effort and to the standards required. (How to set up a quality improvement management system for health promotion work is described in Chapter 4.)

All these functions need to be integrated, for example, strategy and policies must be "owned" by everyone if they are to be effectively implemented. This requires a flexible ("organic") organizational design, based on a number of key principles.

Key principles for designing health-promoting organizations

- First, a *strengthening of teamworking*, and a weakening of formal units (such as functional departments, sections, etc.), narrow specialisms and professional divisions within the organization. Staff will begin to see themselves as primarily members or leaders of a number of teams (or taskforces), with goals and objectives shared by each team. Staff may still have a line manager, but that manager will have more of the characteristics of a facilitator, coach and guide, and fewer of the characteristics of a traditional "boss". Some teams will be created for specific, time-limited projects, others will have continuing responsibilities for particular programmes, services or activities. Each team will require a designated team leader, and for project purposes this will be the "best" person for the job, so that project teams could be led by individuals who are junior in pay and grading to other team members. Teams will often cross departments and professions or even cross organizations, in health alliances. It will be important for team leaders to select the right blend of skills for the task concerned.
- Second, *teams are semi-autonomous*, and responsible for continuously improving the quality of their work. "Right first time" is the operating principle of continuous quality improvement, secured by delegating responsibility for designing appropriate quality improvement systems to the teams, and through ensuring that teams are developed and have the skills and capabilities to perform their tasks. Teams are thus accountable for both the processes and outcomes of their work. They invest time on team building and team development, as well as on the individual development of members, drawing as far as possible on their own resources (6). The autonomy of teams ensures that work is not held up by having to refer decisions up a management hierarchy. It is particularly important for effective joint health working across a number of organizations.
- Third, the management structure above the team level is reduced (flattened). So, a typical organization might have a structure something like the one in Figure 3.1.

Under this sort of arrangement, the Management Board (or its equivalent) is responsible for high-level scanning, for enabling the development of policy and strategy and for agreeing priorities, in the light of policy guidance from higher authorities, such as the NHS Executive, and through agreements based on working in health partnerships with other organizations at local level.

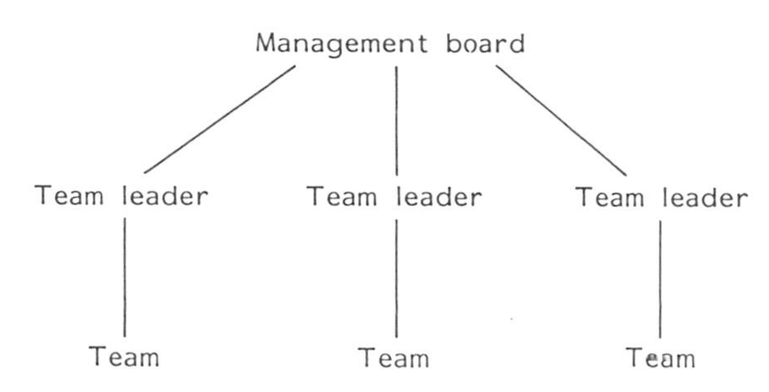

Figure 3.1 A flattened organizational structure

Team leaders include *programme* and *project* coordinators, such as coordinators of "healthy lifestyles" projects, involving joint working by organizations such as NHS Trusts, local authorities, local GPs, schools, workplaces, leisure services, local media and voluntary agencies. Other team leaders provide leadership of continuing *services*, such as health-promoting residential homes for people with mental health problems, or health-promoting maternity services.

For further reading on how to improve organizational effectiveness, see the suggestion at the end of this chapter (7).

DEVELOPING THE HEALTH POTENTIAL OF YOUR STAFF

Operating within a "flattened" organization will bring improved job satisfaction to staff. It will, however, need better identification of the skills, knowledge and attitudes required by staff, and better identification of the means of developing them, so that business objectives are achieved. This will mean prioritizing training and development and taking steps to assure the quality of staff development activities.

For individual members of staff, training and development could bring a number of benefits, such as increased morale and self-esteem, a sharing of problems and development of a shared sense of purpose, reduced stress through the opportunity to reflect and gain a better sense of perspective, a better understanding of the role of others, and increased commitment to the key purposes of the organization. All these benefits are in addition to the actual acquisition of new health development knowledge and skills, which themselves will increase confidence in the ability to change and develop in a fast-changing world!

One of the most obvious ways to develop staff is to provide them with opportunities to attend courses, and there is an increasing range of health promotion and education in-service education and training (INSET) courses available locally, in a range of learning modes such as full-time, part-time, college-based or open learning. For up-to-date details about the availability of courses write to the Health Education Authority or sister organizations in Scotland, Wales and Northern Ireland (8). However, courses are not the only "route to heaven" (becoming better at health promotion and its management) and in many cases are not the most effective alternative to choose from, in a wide range of options (I explain this statement in the next paragraph).

What organizations need to make the best use of their staff is a system which links the individual personal health development plans of staff with the health gain goals, objectives and targets of the organization. Once this is in place it is possible to empower individuals through individual-centred development: enabling individuals to take more responsibility for their own health development and to be more effective in helping the organization to meet its goals. In this way, the benefits to the individual and the benefits to the organization can be simultaneously identified and justify the investment in the development of staff. Then personal development planning can drive the selection of the most appropriate health development responses. (See the section on "Quality management of people" in Chapter 4, for further discussion of this.) The most effective responses bring health development expertise *to* the organization which enables it to develop at the same time as the individuals concerned. (Courses may not be the most effective responses because the person attending a course may develop and change, but the organization may not change, and as a result the person may experience re-entry barriers to using their enhanced abilities.) The most powerful health development responses (which act simultaneously on individuals and the organization) include:

- Health promotion projects and research.
- Secondment to other health-promoting organizations and shadowing more experienced and competent managers or professionals with health promotion experience (see note (13) at the end of Chapter 4 for an explanation of shadowing).
- Health development action learning "sets". (Sets are groups of people who band together and meet regularly to share their learning experiences related to health development "on the job". Quality circles are an example of action learning sets which focus specifically on quality improvement, and these are discussed in Chapter 4.)
- The dissemination of good health promotion practice (this is discussed further in Chapters 4 and 9).

Some of these elements will often be built in to "quality" training courses. Most learning goes on in the workplace, so look at the way you do things—there may be better ways of doing them! Look at what works and also how it can be made to work better. This point is illustrated by the following story.

The importance of learning from experience—a story

A South American tribe kept pigs. One day a grass hut was accidentally burnt down. Inside a pig was tethered, and had come to grief. The smell of the charred meat was delicious and the people tried eating the burnt pig meat and liked it. So they deliberately burnt down grass huts with pigs tethered inside, and ate the meat. Soon they found that they had no huts to live in ...

One of the most important tools for health development, which is immediately accessible to any manager or professional, is to set aside quality time to talk to staff and/or colleagues, both individually, and as teams, in order to learn from workplace experiences.

Assessment of standards of competence (9)

In addition, there is now a new national framework for vocational education and training managed through the National Council for Vocational Qualifications (NCVQ). These changes arose out of both the "Review of Vocational Qualifications in England and Wales" (in 1983) and the government White Paper *Education and Training Together* (10). The new qualification, called National Vocational Qualifications (NVQ), is:

> a statement of competence clearly relevant to work and intended to facilitate entry into, or progression in, employment and further learning, issued to an individual by a recognized awarding body. (11)

A competent person is someone who is able to (12):

- Perform in a specified range of work-related activities to a minimum, specified standard.
- Cope with new working methods, employment patterns and practices insofar as these can be foreseen.
- Transfer their skills from place to place and context to context (within reason).
- Progress to higher NVQ levels more readily than non-competent individuals.

Through the assessment of competencies, employees demonstrate whether they are competent to carry out particular activities. Thus the achievement of competence is based on *assessment*, not on whether a person has followed an agreed curriculum or syllabus of learning, or completed a course. Assessment is the process of gathering evidence about an individual's performance which allows judgements to be made about that person's competence.

There are two phases to the process. First, there is the collection of a portfolio of evidence, which comes from two sources: individual performance and a demonstration of knowledge and understanding. The second phase involves a judgement about whether the evidence meets the standards. Assessment usually takes place in the workplace. The system for making these judgements is through work-based assessors and internal verifiers (provided within employment), monitored by an external verifier, appointed by the awarding body. The competence of the assessors themselves is assessed using the Training and Development Lead Body (TDLB) Units of Competence.

The body responsible for the development of standards of competence in the health and social care field, including those related to health promotion work, is the Occupational Standards Council for Health and Social Care, also referred to as the "Care Sector Consortium" (CSC) (13). In September 1992 the Health Education Authority established a three-year project on "Competencies for Professional Development in Health Education" (14). This is contributing to the work of the Occupational Standards Council for Health and Social Care, in identifying competencies for the health promotion and health education work of a very wide range of professions. Adopting a competence-based approach will bring many benefits and the key ones are summarized in the following box.

The benefits of competence-based assessment and development

1. *Linking training, performance and organizational development*
   The published and agreed occupational standards of competence, which enable occupations as a whole to achieve their key purposes, also enable managers to develop strategic human resource plans for their unit or department. Thus, through a role-mapping exercise, a manager can clarify the competence requirements for the operational work of a department, and therefore the staffing requirements in terms of competencies. Jobs can be redesigned, so that the manager's requirements in terms of clusters of competencies are met. Staff can be developed to meet competence "gaps".

2. *Recruitment and selection*
   The recruitment and selection process is made easier. The job specification is clearer to both interviewers and candidates. Discrimination

continued on next page

continued

is avoided because objective standards are applied. Through identifying "competence gaps" the training needs of new recruits are clear from the outset.

3. *As a basis for staff appraisal*
Because standards of competence are written, published and agreed, with performance criteria for assessment, it is clear what is expected of people in the work role and appraisal is, thus, more focused and more fair.

4. *For identifying and meeting training and development needs*
Within the context of published standards of competence, and performance criteria and evidence, it is possible for managers (and staff) to assess the need for additional experience and/or education and training in order to develop particular competencies. The most appropriate "learning opportunities" can be identified and incorporated into training and development plans.

5. *Improved quality of health promotion work*
The National Occupational Standards for health promotion work will, when developed, provide quality benchmarks for delivery of health promotion. They will be developed within the health and social care sector, by the sector, for the sector.

The competence-based approach helps the manager to exploit the full range of development opportunities, many of which can be provided "on the job" through, for example, coaching, secondment, delegation, critical incident diaries, action learning sets and projects.

All these developments help to minimize the time students are "off the job" for training, provide more flexible training and development opportunities, and also help managers to assure the quality of the work performance of their staff. In a fast-changing world, ensuring that staff are competent to carry out new roles is an increasingly important focus of the work of managers.

The key purpose of all the occupations working in the health and social care sector includes health promotion at its heart. So, for example, the key purpose of health and social care has been defined as (15).

> [to] enable individuals, families, groups and communities to optimize their health and social well-being balancing their respective needs with those of society as a whole and the resources available.

This key purpose can be broken down into a number of functions and thence into the competencies required for each function. With respect to health promotion, the competencies required are about working with people to promote health in many different situations with a variety of different aims. To do this, knowledge of particular methods and special skills are necessary. These are not necessarily exclusive to health promotion work, but they are the core competencies of health promotion. ("Core competencies" is a term used to refer to those which are common to a number of different occupations.)

The standards of competence for work in health promotion are not yet published. However, in the meantime there is still much benefit to be gained by identifying the health promotion role of staff. For a current analysis of the core competency areas of health promotion work, see Ewles and Simnett (16). They identify six clusters of competencies necessary for health promotion work:

- Managing, planning and evaluating.
- Communicating.
- Educating.
- Marketing and publicizing.
- Facilitating and networking.
- Influencing policy and practice.

You can analyse the health promotion role of your staff by undertaking a role-mapping exercise, through considering how health promotion contributes to each of their functions. Examples are provided in the following box.

Examples of mapping the health promotion role

1. You are the manager of a ward in a hospital. The health promotion roles of your staff include:
   - Communication and education which contributes to treatment: if giving treatment to patients is part of the work of your staff, the health education elements may include explaining why the treatment is necessary, what the member of staff is doing and what it will feel like.
   - Communicating and educating through health information: other staff may be involved in designing leaflets to inform patients, and their relatives and carers, about their condition and how they can play an active part in recovery or management of the condition.
   - Managing, planning and evaluating during the implementation of health promotion policies and regulations: your staff will be responsible for implementing regulations and policies designed to protect or maintain the health of patients and of staff (such as food hygiene regulations, policies to control the spread of infections, to

continued on next page

continued

prevent the misuse of alcohol and drugs, to promote healthy eating, on HIV/AIDS, and no-smoking policies).

- Influencing policy and practice through health promotion research: some staff may be involved in research and development work in health promotion, for example through profiling the health promotion needs of patients.
- Facilitating and networking: some staff may be concerned with facilitating the development of students on placement in your ward. Most staff will belong to networks, such as branches of professional associations, which are concerned with spreading good health promotion practice.
- Marketing and publicizing: some staff may be concerned with publicizing services offered by the ward to relatives or to other groups in the community (for example, a paediatric ward may wish to publicize "open days" when parents and children and local schools can come and see for themselves what happens when a child stays in hospital).

2. You are the manager of a primary health care facilitator (17). The role of a primary care facilitator is wholly in health promotion work, and includes:
   - Facilitating practice nurses in introducing systematic screening programmes, for example, to detect the major risk factors for arterial disease. This will include communicating and educating, for example through explaining why the screening service is necessary and providing training in how to approach health education with patients, including how to help patients to change health-related behaviours. Educating and training the practice nurse in managing, planning and evaluating will also be necessary, for example, on how to carry out the health checks and record information.
   - Facilitating improved standards of marketing by practices of the health promotion services they have on offer, for example, through enabling links with the local mass media.
   - Communicating with, and educating and training, receptionists in their role in managing, planning and evaluating, for example, through explaining how to keep records and operate the recall system.
   - Networking through gathering and providing health promotion information to practices, for example about wider health promotion programmes to which a practice could contribute.
   - Influencing policy and practice through:—Encouraging and supporting health promotion research and development work within a practice.
     - — Advising on health promotion quality improvement schemes, for example on how to evaluate health promotion activities or on how to set quality standards for health promotion work.
     - — Advising a practice on how to design and implement health promotion policies and health development strategies, which will ensure that it is becoming a health-promoting organization.

   Here, the health promotion is aimed at other professions, rather than the public, with the purpose of "facilitating" the other professions in providing health promotion services to the public.

You can use the information gathered through such a role-mapping exercise as the starting point for a review of the health promotion performance of your staff, as a basis for individual performance review (appraisal), for identifying their training and development needs and making a training and development plan.

"COMMISSIONING": FORMULATING HEALTH STRATEGY AND PROGRAMMES

> New growths insensibly bud upwards to fill each vacated place; unforseen accidents hinder intentions, and old plans are forgotten.
>
> Thomas Hardy: *Tess of the d'Urbervilles*, Ch. 36.

The White Papers *Working for Patients* and *Caring for People* and the subsequent National Health Service and Community Care Act 1990 (18) heralded a turning-point for the NHS. There is now a climate of "managerialism" with an emphasis on getting results and providing value for money. The search is on for measurable outcomes—tangible evidence that the vast sums of public money invested in health and social care are actually doing good. These outcomes are health benefits or "health gain" (I have already provided a definition of health gain in Chapter 1). The emphasis is on achieving improved *health and well-being*, rather than on just providing health *services* or social *care*. The separation between "purchasers" (sometimes alternatively referred to as "commissioners") and "providers" means that the purchasers (commissioners) are now responsible for developing strategies to achieve health gain for the population they serve (19).

A local health gain strategy will be the most important vehicle for ensuring that the national strategy for health is implemented at local level (20). Any health gain strategy will be based on the "health gain spiral" which I described in Chapter 1 (stage 1—assess needs; stage 2—plan; stage 3—do; stage 4—evaluate; stage 5—review). It must address a number of key issues, including:

1. What are the key results areas for commissioning?

   To answer this question will require a thorough analysis of:

   - Needs for health promotion, treatment, care and rehabilitation, based on evidence about why particular conditions or issues are a priority area for local commissioning, in terms of how big each problem is, and what the major risk factors are.
   - What effective interventions are available to increase health gain, related to each of the priorities, and what programmes are currently purchased and provided? (This may require a review of the effectiveness of current provisions.)

- What are the views of local people? (A useful tool for debating priorities is provided in a recent HEA publication on *Promoting Physical Activity*) (21).

2. What is the agreed health gain strategy?
   - The agreed strategy will ideally set out an *integrated* strategy for health promotion, treatment (when relevant), rehabilitation and care, but in practice these may be addressed by *separate* strategies, which will then require arrangements for integration (see point 4 below).
   - The measurable targets for health gain which the commissioning authority has adopted will require specification in a *strategic health plan*. (I discuss health strategies and targets in more detail in Chapter 6.)
   - The plan will also include detailed specifications for the actions required to achieve the targets, first in terms of broad *programme (key results) areas* (for example, through specification of plans related to a coherent set of health promotion, treatment, care and rehabilitation services directed towards an identified health problem such as HIV/AIDS), and then in terms of *services, projects and activities* to be commissioned as contributors to each programme area.
   - The plan will specify costs, inputs, quality standards and quality improvement systems and mechanisms for monitoring, evaluating and reviewing the programmes and the overall health gain strategy.
3. What are the implications of the health strategy for all those concerned?

   The strategic health plan will also spell out the implications of the strategy for each of the various players, such as:
   - Primary care.
   - Hospital providers.
   - Community providers.
   - Employers, and commercial organizations.
   - Educational institutions, schools, etc.
   - Commissioning health authorities.
   - GP fundholders.
   - Voluntary organizations and non-statutory bodies.
   - Local government.
   - User groups/ Community Health Council.
   - Ambulance services.
   - Alliances for health.
   - Other agents and agencies.
4. How will the health strategy be integrated, so that a concerted effort is achieved?

   A key feature of the strategic health plan will be the arrangements for coordination, cooperation and collaboration between the key players involved in designing and implementing the strategy, through:

- Arrangements for *joint* commissioning by health authorities/health commissions and local authorities and other agencies.
- Mechanisms for links between this strategy and other local health and social care strategies (for example, community care strategies, healthy city strategies, local authority strategies to improve environmental conditions or "green" plans).
- Mechanisms for links between programme areas, in order to achieve synergy and avoid duplication of efforts. (*Synergy* occurs when the combined effects of two or more interventions produces a greater impact than could be achieved by each intervention undertaken separately. For example, physical activity is important in the promotion of mental health and well-being; the prevention and rehabilitation of coronary heart disease and strokes; the prevention and reduction of obesity; the prevention of osteoporosis and the prevention of accidents. A programme to promote physical activity could therefore contribute to separate programmes in all these areas.)
- It could also highlight the management arrangements at provider level, such contract agreements, grant and partnership arrangements, and the mechanisms to encourage effective communication from both top to bottom and bottom to top, and horizontally, across and within partner organizations.

Formulating such a health gain strategy involves gathering a great deal of information, both on the size and nature of health problems and on whether effective and acceptable responses are available. With respect to health promotion, or to the balance between health promotion and treatment and care, such a comprehensive needs assessment cannot be attempted in every area simultaneously, and there has to be some way of determining which subjects should be investigated as a priority, and in what depth. The factors to consider are set out in the following box.

Criteria to use when deciding whether a comprehensive health needs assessment is necessary

- The issue or condition has a big impact on health (morbidity and mortality), i.e. the issue has serious consequences.
- It is a major consumer of resources.
- Effective measures are available for both health promotion, treatment and rehabilitation and care, and it is important to determine the right balance between them.
- The issue or condition is a matter of local concern, for example, to GPs or to local people.

Health needs assessment requires considerable skills and must therefore be carried out by competent people, including public health physicians, epidemiologists, statisticians, health promotion specialists and health economists. It can confirm or refute an impression of need gained from anecdotes by health and social care and other workers. How to carry out a full health needs assessment is beyond the scope of this book, but further reading is suggested at the end of this chapter (22).

The NHS is not yet equipped to take the approach to commissioning which I have just described. Health gain remains a largely theoretical concept and one with which commissioners often do not truly engage (23). This is because of the failure to address the management development, organizational development, professional development and personal development needs related to *The Health of the Nation*. This book is one contribution to fill that gap.

Rapid appraisal

Rapid participatory appraisal is a research method which was originally developed for use in developing countries but is now being increasingly used in the UK to provide information which will assist both in the commissioning and providing of services to meet health and social needs of local populations. It can be used in this context to gain insight into a community's own perspective on its health needs and to translate these into action. It is also a way of establishing a continuing relationship between service purchasers, providers and local communities.

It involves researchers drawn from the local community and uses a strategy of returning to the community to confirm findings, and to explore the implications of those findings for the local community and for service providers.

Community profiling is similar in approach to rapid appraisal and is being used in relation to a variety of local public services including housing, social and health care, urban regeneration and economic development, and leisure and recreation. For further reading on rapid appraisal and community profiling, see the suggestions at the end of this chapter (24).

The key steps for conducting a rapid appraisal are (25):

1. Decide what information is needed (this should be relevant and minimal).
2. Decide how you will obtain the information (e.g. from existing documents, interviews with key informants, observations).

3. Decide who should collect the information (involve the community and partner agencies).
4. Analyse the information (this should be rapid but checked against "common sense" and available health statistics).
5. Check the findings with key informants and local knowledge.
6. Select priorities for action.
7. Plan the actions and outcomes.
8. Monitor the plan—activities and quality.
9. Evaluate.

One recent UK example of using rapid appraisal is in Dumbidykes, a small council estate in Edinburgh, where six priority areas for health development were identified. The approach led to an improved multidisciplinary way of working and complemented quantitative methods of assessing need (26).

"PROVIDING": WORKING TOWARDS BETTER HEALTH IN YOUR OWN SETTING (27)

There are many ways that managers and professionals working in "provider" agencies can be involved in a health promotion strategy. You could initiate it; you could encourage someone else to initiate it; you could "champion" it; you could "sign up" to it; you could communicate it. Here, I focus on two aspects: how you can work in your own setting and how you can work together with other managers, professionals and other organizations. The first step is to find out what is already going on and then get started in your own setting. How to do this is described in the following box.

Finding out what is going on in health promotion and getting started

1. Find out about local plans from your NHS Specialist Health Promotion Service (the role of NHS Specialist Health Promotion Services is described in the next section of this chapter).
2. Network with other organizations, who are involved in health promotion work, to find out what they are doing.
3. Gain staff support through briefing your staff and colleagues on the concept and characteristics of health-promoting organizations, perhaps getting help from your local specialist health promotion service to do this.

continued on next page

continued

4. Involve staff/colleagues in finding out (reviewing/auditing) what is currently going on in your own unit, department or business. Look for:
   - Policies on smoking, healthy eating, sensible drinking, promotion of physical activity, promotion of mental health and prevention of stress, prevention of the spread of infections, HIV/AIDS, equal opportunities and occupational health.
   - *Procedures* and *protocols* related to health, hygiene and safety.
   - *Management practices* to support the health of staff (such as subsidizing the cost of staff joining local health and fitness clubs and the provision of crèche facilities or play schemes, or the provision of counselling to cope with stress).
   - *Practices related to promoting the health of patients* (for example, through the after-care provided after discharge from hospital).
   - *Environmental measures* (such as the provision of fitness facilities on site, a hospital Trim-trail, showering facilities for staff who wish to exercise in the lunch hour).
   - Special promotional events such as exhibitions, participation in national no-smoking day, conferences.
   - *Participation in local, national or international programmes.* (Please note: you may wish to read Chapters 4 and 5 before you do this.)
5. Involve staff in analysing the findings.
6. Publicize your findings with potential partners (community groups, local authorities, voluntary groups, academic institutions, service user groups), perhaps through the local media, or a conference, or through focus groups to get their active participation.
7. Designate a manager to coordinate the health promotion programmes and activities of your unit/department.
8. Assess the needs for health promotion (for example, of staff, patients, visitors and students) and develop an action plan, in partnership with them and with other local organizations, using techniques such as rapid appraisal.

WORKING IN HEALTH PARTNERSHIPS

Health promotion activities are often delivered at a very local level, to particular neighbourhoods, or to particular groups of people within particular localities. The practitioners who deliver the health promotion at operational level are many and varied, including primary health care teams, teachers, social workers, pharmacists, probation officers, police officers, dietitians, environmental health officers, fitness advisors, volunteers working for voluntary organizations, occupational health staff, managers in local businesses, trades union staff, restaurateurs, and leisure services staff (28). Those responsible for providing and improving "healthy" facilities and amenities, such as traffic-calming schemes, swimming baths and cycleways, are all health promotion providers, as are manufacturers and retailers who market "healthy" products such as healthy food and safe toys. Without a strategic approach to the design and delivery of activities much effort could fail to "hit the mark", with duplication, waste and a failure to be effective as a consequence.

In addition, the work within localities needs to be integrated with the strategic health plans of commissioners, whether these are a health commission or a strategic health alliance, for example, a "Green" Cities Partnership, or an alliance on a particular issue, such as "Heart Health". Often, the health promotion delivered within a locality will also be linked to initiatives taken at national level, for example initiatives by the Health Education Authority, or the Department of Health, as part of *The Health of the Nation* (or corresponding strategies in other parts of the UK).

The agency which has a lead role in enabling all these links to be made is the local NHS Specialist Health Promotion Department, which could be part of a Health Commissioning Agency, or part of an NHS Trust, or, indeed, a "freestanding" agency. We now move on to describe the work of specialist Health Promotion Departments in more detail (many local authorities also have specialist health promotion, or health development, sections).

The role of Specialist Health Promotion Services

You can expect your local Specialist Health Promotion Services to do some or all of the following:

- Provide consultancy, advice, training, information and resources to support local health promotion work, whether it is undertaken by NHS staff or by others, such as schoolteachers, employers, those responsible for environmental improvements, voluntary agencies and many others.
- Provide help with policy development, whether it is a health promotion policy (such as a food and health policy) for use in your own setting, or to examine the impact of other policies (such as transport policies) on health.
- Coordinate local activities so that organizations and groups are aligning themselves strategically to maximize health promotion opportunities.
- Support managers and planners with meeting *Health of the Nation* targets (or corresponding targets in other parts of the UK), including help with setting local targets and measuring progress towards them.
- Help managers and professionals with making links with the community (for example, Specialist Health Promotion Services may implement community health development projects for particular localities, and may therefore have considerable experience in this field).

- Help managers and professionals with networking and enabling health promotion activities to happen (for example, helping you to make links with local media).
- Help managers and professionals with managing, planning and evaluating health promotion activities.
- Provide a range of health promotion programmes related to key areas (such as HIV/AIDS and sexual health), key settings (such as health in the workplace) and key target groups (such as young people).
- Provide small grants to local groups wanting to develop specific health promotion activities.

Historically, many Specialist Health Promotion Services started by providing resources (such as leaflets, audiovisual aids and posters) for local health promoters to use, as one of their main functions. Most services still include this function, but have evolved into a much more strategic role, functioning as negotiators and enablers between and within organizations, in order to ensure that the best use is made of all local resources for improving the health of local populations.

Some Specialist Health Promotion Services have recently produced a "Statement of Intent" or a "Mission Statement" which provides strategic direction for the service. For example, the Mission Statement of Health First (the main provider of specialist health promotion in Lambeth, Lewisham and Southwark) is (29):

> Health First works for positive health in the boroughs of Lambeth, Lewisham and Southwark by improving the health of their people, reducing health inequalities and encouraging local communities to value their health. The service encourages the promotion of physical, mental, emotional and social well-being as well as the reduction of illness, disease and premature death.

Health promotion services are thus "health development agencies", which focus on developing health promoters, health-promoting organizations, health alliances, and on community health development.

The role of NHS Trusts

If you are a manager with an NHS Trust you may have a range of different things in your contract which are related to health promotion:

- If yours is a Community Trust, you may be concerned with developing the role of health visitors to enable them to work in different ways, for example as public health workers or as advocates. In some localities, for example, health visitors have been developed to act as public health nurses, who develop strategies to promote the health of the population at neighbourhood level.

- If yours is an Acute Trust, you may be developing guidelines on the standards of written information which patients receive before discharge, or you may be developing guidelines on how hospitals can consult with client groups.

In Stockport, for example, "Guidelines for Producing Written Information" was launched in July 1993, and nurses, business managers and heads of departments have been briefed about the guidelines (30). A copy has been sent to every ward, clinic and department in the district and managers are responsible for ensuring that staff have easy access to the guidelines.

Basically, there are three key aspects to the work of NHS Trusts related to their health promotion role:

- NHS Trusts as service providers.
- NHS Trusts as employers.
- NHS Trusts as partners with other agencies in the community.

Agreements with purchasers often spell out the provider role. An example is given in the following box.

Example of an agreement on health promotion between a purchaser and a provider

Stockport Health Authority has the following Local Charter Standard agreed between provider and purchaser related to health promotion and illness prevention:

1. Each Directorate within the Provider Units will have a designated senior member of staff responsible for coordinating health promotion activity and standards.
2. The Provider Units will operate the Stockport Health Authority's health promotion policies on smoking, alcohol, food and health, and equal opportunities, all of which will be reviewed annually.
3. Each Provider Unit will ensure that two people from each ward/clinic/ paramedical group are trained in health education techniques.
4. All written patient education material will follow the guidelines agreed by Stockport Health Authority.
5. The two most common treatment/therapies in each ward/clinic/ paramedical group will have written information for patients/carers.

There are also a number of national, and international, initiatives which can provide a focus for the health promotion work of NHS Trusts, and I describe some of these in Chapter 8.

Health promotion projects initiated by hospitals

An increasing number of health promotion projects are being initiated by hospitals, often in partnership with local NHS Specialist Health Promotion Services. One recent innovative example is related to the promotion of continence and is described in the following box (31).

Example of a hospital health promotion project

Time for dignity

Staff at Seacroft Hospital in Leeds have produced individual care plans for elderly mentally ill patients who have continence problems, through assessing the time of day when patients most needed help. Continence aids have also been measured to make sure that they are suitable for each individual. Within two weeks of implementing the care plans, incontinence levels—and the resulting distress—dropped noticeably; the patients' dignity and self-esteem increased, and staff attitudes to continence management changed.

The role of primary health care

The new GP contracts have expanded the role of GPs in health promotion. However, the efficacy of the government's current health promotion package for primary care, based on multifactorial risk factor assessment and lifestyle intervention, is questionable (32). The British family heart study, in a randomized controlled trial of nurse-led screening for cardiovascular risk factors and lifestyle intervention on families in general practices in towns throughout Britain, achieved at most an overall 12% reduction in coronary risk and concluded that the health promotion package in primary care cannot be justified in its present form (33). Another recent randomized controlled study of the effectiveness of health checks conducted by nurses in primary care concluded that general health checks by nurses are ineffective in helping smokers to stop smoking, but they do help patients to modify their diet (34). The lack of effectiveness of health checks in promoting smoking cessation contrasts with the effectiveness of trials of nicotine patches in general practice. These researchers conclude that practice nurses may be more effectively used with patients at established high risk, for example to improve the management of patients with hypertension and high cholesterol concentration.

These studies should not be interpreted as casting doubt on GPs' opportunistic use of routine consultations for health promotion. There is also growing evidence that brief interventions by primary care workers with people who are ready to change their lifestyles are effective (35). (For further discussion of brief, effective interventions to change patients' health behaviours and lifestyles, and of the pivotal role of the GP in health and health promotion strategy, including a discussion on the future role of primary health care, see Chapter 9.) The evidence therefore suggests that the new contract imposed on GPs is both ineffective and unethical. Better approaches to health promotion in primary health care are available and the contracts should be changed.

The National Association of Patient Participation (NAPP) supports Patient Participation Groups in GP surgeries and health centres (36). For further information on health promotion in primary care, see the suggestion in the note at the end of the chapter (37).

An activity you could undertake: identifying which teams in your organization need health development

Using the categories suggested, and others if necessary, identify all the teams you are involved with in your organization, and prioritize their needs for health development using relevant criteria, such as:

- Teams which have the best potential for health development.
- Teams whose health promotion performance or morale is low.
- Teams whose work is vital to the achievement of the key purpose of your organization.
- Teams whose members are ready to develop (for example, teams committed to the concept of health-promoting organizations or multi-agency teams already working on aspects of health promotion).
- Teams who have resources available for health development.

Rank each team for all the criteria you consider are appropriate and relevant.

Suggestions for categories of teams

- *The top team*: the senior management group or board responsible for policy and strategy.
- *A management group*: a group of managers (for example, a group of programme managers, each responsible for their own programme area, who need to ensure that their work is integrated).
- *A programme management team*: a team responsible for a defined key results area, involving substantial and long-term work. This team may continue to operate for many years and will need to adapt its role and

continued on next page

continued

membership as circumstances change. It will often include members from a number of partner organizations, each with their own agendas.

- A project team: a group of people responsible for achieving a defined objective. The team members may report to various managers, perhaps in different organizations. The team has a defined life expectancy.
- *A service team*: a group which interacts directly with service users and is responsible for delivery of a defined service. The team includes a service manager or team leader and staff from different professions and disciplines who are all involved in service provisions (for example, a ward team in a hospital).
- A professional team: a group who all belong to the same profession and are responsible for the same function, but work with different groups of clients, and need to ensure their professional development and peer support/supervision.

Finally, consider what contribution you could make to the health development of these teams, and what other sources of help may be available to them. (You may wish to read the section on "How to build health-promoting teams in Chapter 7, at this point.)

Questions you could ask yourself

Consider how you need to improve your own health promotion management performance, through asking yourself:

- What are the main areas I need to improve?
- What sources of help are available to me (list all the sources for each area in which you need to improve)?
- What is my action plan for improving?
- When will I review my progress (on what date) and what are the appropriate criteria to assess my improvement?

NOTES, REFERENCES AND FURTHER READING

(1) McGregor, D. (1960) *The Human Side of Enterprise* Maidenhead: McGraw-Hill International.

(2) Townend, A. (1991) *Developing Assertiveness*. London: Routledge.

For self-help guides which explain how the principles of behavioural psychology can be used to increase control over your own behaviour, see:

Watson, D.L. and Tharp, R.G. (4th edn, 1985) *Self-directed Behaviour: Self-modification for Personal Adjustment*. Monterey, CA: Brooks/Cole.

Simon, S.B. (1989) *Change Your Life Right Now! Breaking Down the Barriers to Success*. Wellingborough: Thorsons.

(3) Some of the key skills required for managing health promotion are discussed in:

Ewles, L. and Simnett, I. (3rd edn, 1995) *Promoting Health: A Practical Guide.* London: Scutari Press. Ch. 7.

(4) The unit written by Glenn MacDonald, "Reflecting on the Management Process", in *Management Competencies for Health Gain,* which is part of the *Managing Health Improvement Project* (MAHIP) open learning materials, looks in detail at the personal and interpersonal issues which are likely to impinge on the effectiveness of health promotion management. For further information about the availability of these materials, see note (8) in Chapter 1.

See also:

Reeves, T. (1994) *Managing Effectively: Developing Yourself Through Experience.* Oxford: Butterworth-Heinemann, in association with the Institute of Management.

See also the suggestions in note (11), in Chapter 1.

(5) A *policy* is a formal statement or procedure within organizations (including government). A *health policy* is one which gives priority to health or which recognizes health goals. It may involve health services or other sectors which affect health, such as local government.

The *strategy* of an organization consists of a mission, goals, objectives and targets, unique to that organization.

(6) For an introduction to team theory and to activities which will help build teams in health promotion settings, see:

Rolls, E. (1992) *Team Development: A Manual of Facilitation for Health Educators and Health Promoters.* London: Health Education Authority.

(7) For a recent publication which explores ways in which management standards can be used to enhance organizational processes, see:

NHS Training Division (1994) *Using Management Standards to Improve Organizational Effectiveness.* Bristol: NHSTD.

(8) England: Health Education Authority, Hamilton House, Mabledon Place, London WC1H 9TX. Telephone: 0171 383 3833.

Northern Ireland: Health Promotion Agency for Northern Ireland, 18 Ormeau Avenue, Belfast BT2 8HS. Telephone: 01232 311611.

Scotland: Health Education Board for Scotland, Woodburn House, Canaan Lane, Edinburgh EH10 4SG. Telephone: 0131 447 8044.

Wales: Health Promotion Wales, Ffynnon-las, Ty Glas Avenue, Llanishen, Cardiff CF4 5DZ. Telephone: 01222 752 222.

(9) Manpower Services Commission and the Department of Education and Science (April 1983) *Review of Vocational Qualifications in England and Wales.* London: DES.

HM Government White Paper (1986) *Education and Training Together*. London: HMSO. Cm. 9823.

(10) National Council for Vocational Qualifications (1989) quoted in: National Health Service Training Directorate (1992) *NVQ's: Getting Started*. Bristol: NHSTD. p. 27.

(11) Johnson, C. and Blinkhorn, S. (1992) Validating NVQ Assessment. *Competence and Assessment*, issue 20. Sheffield: Department of Employment. p. 12.

(12) This section is based on information provided by Liz Rolls, the HEA Competencies Project Coordinator.

(13) Care Sector Consortium (Occupational Standards Council for Health and Social Care), Rooms 29–35, 14 Russell Square, London WC1B 5EP. Telephone: 0171 972 8314/5.

For further information on National Occupational Standards, including case studies of how these are being used across the UK, see the leaflet and case study booklet available from the CSC, at the address above.

(14) The HEA Competencies Project Coordinator is based at Cheltenham and Gloucester College of Higher Education, PO Box 220, The Park Campus, The Park, Cheltenham, Glos GL50 2QF. Telephone: 01242 532874.

(15) This definition is used by Prime Research and Development Ltd in draft material produced for the Care Sector Consortium, May 1994.

(16) See:

Ewles, L. and Simnett, I. (3rd edn, 1995) *Promoting Health: A Practical Guide*. London: Scutari Press. Ch. 2.

(17) *Facilitation* is enabling people to do something for themselves, through support and encouragement, rather than doing it for them. In health promotion work, it refers to helping people to improve their own and/or other people's health.

(18) HM Government White Paper (1989) *Working for Patients*. London: HMSO.

HM Government White Paper (1989) *Caring for People*. London: HMSO.

(19) I describe what is meant by commissioners and providers in note (13) of Chapter 1. In the health services, the purchasers are health authorities, FHSAs, or health commissions formed by mergers of these agencies, and GP fundholders, and the providers are hospital and community health services, many of which are now NHS Trusts and managerially independent of their parent authorities, and primary health care agents and agencies.

(20) How to develop a local strategy and a commissioning plan, related to the promotion of physical activity, is discussed in detail in:

Health Education Authority (1995) *Promoting Physical Activity: Guidance for Commissioners, Purchasers and Providers*. London: HEA.

(21) Health Education Authority (1995) *Promoting Physical Activity: Guidance for Commissioners, Purchasers and Providers*. London: HEA.

(22) The volume entitled 'Needs Assessment for Health Improvement and Health Gain, which is part of the *Managing Health Improvement Project* (MAHIP) open learning material, was written by Peter Brambleby, Ina Simnett and Myrtle Summerly, and describes concepts of need and approaches to needs assessment in detail. For information about the availability of these materials, see note (8) in Chapter 1.

Identifying health promotion needs and priorities is discussed in:

Ewles, L. and Simnett, I. (3rd edn, 1995) *Promoting Health: A Practical Guide.* London: Scutari Press. Ch 5.

See also:

NHS Management Executive (1991) *Assessing Health Care Needs: A DHA Project Discussion Paper.* London: NHSME.

Mooney, G.H., Russell, E.M. and Weir, R.D. (1986) *Choices for Health Care.* London: Macmillan.

Donaldson, C. and Mooney, G. (1991) Needs assessment, priority setting and contracts for health care: an economic view. *British Medical Journal* **303**: 1029–1030.

(23) Hunter, D. and Alderslade, R. (1994) Public health management: outward bound. *Health Service Journal* **104** (5426): 22–24.

(24) Annett, H. and Rifkin, S. (1988) *Guidelines for Rapid Appraisal to Assess Community Health Needs: A Focus on Health Improvement for Low Income Areas.* Geneva: World Health Organization.

Burton, P. (1993) *Community Profiling: A Guide to Identifying Local Needs.* Bristol: School for Advanced Urban Studies, University of Bristol.

Hawtin, M., Percy-Smith, J., Hughes, G. with Foreman, A. (1994) *Community Profiling: Auditing Social Needs.* Milton Keynes: Open University Press.

Ong, B. and Humphris, G. (1994) Prioritising needs in urban communities: the rapid appraisal methodology in health. In: Popay, J. and Williams G. (eds), *Researching the People's Health: Social Research in Health Care.* London: Routledge.

(25) These steps are based on steps for participatory rapid assessment described in:

Health Education Authority (1995) *Promoting Physical Activity: Guidance for Commissioners, Purchasers and Providers.* London: HEA.

(26) Murray, S.A., Tapson, J., Turnbull, L. *et al.* (1994) Listening to local voices: adapting rapid appraisal to assess health and social needs in general practice. *British Medical Journal*, **308**: 698–700.

(27) This section, and the following section, "Working in partnerships", are partly based on information in the volume entitled *The Design and Implementation of Strategies for Health Improvement*, which is part of the *Managing Health Improvement Project* (MAHIP) open learning material. For further information

on the role of purchasers and providers in health gain strategies, see this volume. For information about the availability of this material, see note (8) in Chapter 1.

(28) The role of health promoters is discussed in detail in:

Ewles, L. and Simnett, I. (3rd edn, 1995) *Promoting Health: A Practical Guide.* London: Scutari Press. Ch. 4.

(29) This Mission Statement is part of the Statement of Intent for Health First, copies of which can be obtained from Health First, Mary Sheridan House, 15 St Thomas Street, London SE1 9RY. Telephone: 0171 955 4366.

(30) Copies of the "Guidelines for the Production of Written Materials" can be obtained from Lucy Hamer, Stockport Health Authority, Centre for Health Promotion, 188 Buxton Road, Stockport, Cheshire SK2 7AE. Telephone: 0161 456 0119.

(31) This example is based on information in *Health Promoting Hospitals,* No. 1, Summer 1994. p. 5.

Health Promoting Hospitals is the magazine produced by the Preston Health Promoting Hospital Project. For further information about this project contact the Information Line: Preston Health Promotion Unit, Sharoe Green Hospital, Watling Street Road, Fulwood, Preston PR2 4DX. Telephone: 01772 711223.

(32) Stott, N. (1994) Screening for cardiovascular risk in general practice: blanket health promotion is a waste of resources. *British Medical Journal* **308**: 285–286.

(33) Wood, D.A., Kinmonth, A.L, Pyke, S.D.M. and Thompson, S.G. (1994) Randomised controlled trial evaluating cardiovascular screening and intervention in general practice: principal results of British family heart study. *British Medical Journal* **308**: 313–320.

(34) Muir, J., Mant, D., Jones L. and Yudkin, P. (1994) Effectiveness of health checks conducted by nurses in primary care: results of the OXCHECK study after one year. *British Medical Journal,* **308**: 308–312.

(35) Rollnick, S., Kinnersley, P. and Stott, N. (1993) Methods of helping patients with behaviour change. *British Medical Journal* **307**: 188–190.

(36) A starter pack for setting up a patient participation group is available from NAPP, 50 Wallasey Village, Wallasey L45 3NT.

(37) The role of primary health care and community health services is discussed in detail in the material on health promotion work in this setting, which forms part of the *Managing Health Improvement Project* (MAHIP) material. For information about the availability of this material, see note (8) in Chapter 1.

CHAPTER 4 Quality improvement and health development

Summary

This chapter addresses how to improve the quality of health promotion work through designing and implementing a strategy for continuous quality improvement which focuses on three key dimensions: management quality, professional quality, and "people power" (involving local people in defining and delivering high quality health promotion activities). It starts by discussing what is meant by quality improvement in relation to health promotion and why it is important to *manage* for quality. It then looks at what are the basic elements of a quality improvement management system and provides some information on how local people could become more involved in health promotion. The next section makes some suggestions about how "providers" could get started. The following section continues by examining how to specify for quality and provides examples of health promotion specifications, including standards. This is followed by a discussion on how best to manage people, why this is an important aspect of quality management, and what skills are required. It then moves on to consider the role of managers and professionals in professional development and spreading good practice. It ends with a suggested activity, which you could undertake, in order to improve your skills in peer supervision and support, and some questions you could ask yourself, in order to identify how to move forward with quality improvement.

QUALITY IMPROVEMENT AND HEALTH PROMOTION WORK

People are often mystified by all the jargon and hype associated with quality. I discuss the meaning of some important terms used, related to quality, in the note at the end of the chapter (1). The confusion created by the lack of general agreement on the meaning of terms can be "disempowering", so it is important first to carefully consider the meaning of terms, and also to establish what are the key principles to use when working for improved quality. By quality I simply mean looking at the nature of a service, policy or intervention, and assessing how "good" it is when judged against a number of criteria. The basis of working for quality improvement in health promotion activities is actually fairly straightforward. There are three key dimensions of quality which must be addressed (2):

- *Management quality*: the quality of the management of health promotion.
- *Professional quality*: the quality of the performance of the health promoters who directly provide health promotion to members of the public.
- *Participation by local people*: the quality of participation by local people so that health promotion activities meet their requirements.

Quality improvement in relation to health promotion is thus about:

1. Having good management systems and procedures which will ensure that you are succeeding in continually improving the quality of your work.
2. Spreading good health promotion practices across all the professions and occupations who play a part.
3. Ensuring that the health promotion activities meet stakeholder requirements. (Stakeholders are all those people and agencies with an interest in the outcomes.) This requires genuine engagement with the public through informed debate.

The most important thing to bear in mind is that the systems required to address these three dimensions must involve repeating a cyclical process (a quality cycle) in order to be effective.

The manager is ultimately responsible for ensuring that effective quality improvement systems are in place, but it involves a collective effort and in this chapter I discuss how managers, professionals and the public all play a part in managing for quality in health promotion work.

SETTING UP A SYSTEM FOR MANAGING THE QUALITY OF HEALTH PROMOTION WORK

"Quality" management is about ensuring that activities are cost-effective (i.e. provide value for money) and make efficient use of resources, within the policies set by the management board of an organization (or its equivalent), or by "higher" authorities, for example by a health commissioning agency or the Department of Health.

There are a number of reasons why it is important to focus on managing for high-quality health promotion work. These include:

- *To prioritize and make choices which ensure the best possible use of resources* through, for example, being able to assess which of a number of alternative ways of achieving the same outcomes involve the minimum inputs in terms of time, staff and money or how to ensure the maximum return on a fixed investment of resources (*cost effectiveness*).

- *To improve quality in specific key areas* through focusing on important aspects of health promotion, such as how to extend access to more people, or how to improve health promotion methods, or how to increase user satisfaction, or how to improve communication.
- *To win contracts* through demonstrating the value of health promotion work to purchasers.
- *To assess whether activities are ethically sound* by, for example, demonstrating that benefits for some people are not gained at the expense of losses for others, and that anxiety and stress which may be associated with some interventions are kept to an acceptable minimum.
- *To ensure maximum health gain*: the maximum possible improvement in the health of local people is the goal of health promotion work (*effectiveness*).

Essentially, what you need to do to have a "quality" health promotion management system is to:

1. *Identify quality needs and agree priorities for quality*: each stakeholder (individuals and groups with an interest in the quality of health promotion work) may have a different view about what are the most important aspects of quality. It is therefore essential, right from the start, to identify and reconcile, as far as possible, these different viewpoints. This can be done through being open about the differences and facilitating discussion, in order to identify areas of agreement on what is important and what is acceptable. The bottom line is that quality health promotion must meet the requirements of the local population or group of people concerned. This may not be the same as the needs of *service users*, because the *non-users* need to become involved in health promotion, and these may be the people with the greatest needs. (For example, those people who are not registered with a GP may be the people in a locality with the greatest needs.)
2. *Develop and supervise your staff*: support staff so that they take responsibility for quality of health promotion.
3. *Regularly review and improve specifications*: tighten up on the health promotion elements of specifications for everything important, from your mission, to planning, implementation and evaluation procedures.
4. *Introduce quality assurance systems*: identify critical aspects of your health promotion services and introduce systems to prevent problems arising in these areas (this is usually referred to as "quality assurance").

5. *Introduce quality control systems*: make regular checks which show that you are carrying out agreed health promotion policies and procedures correctly and consistently, and that any problems are identified and corrected (this is usually referred to as "quality control"). Ensure that your health promotion specifications are being achieved, through evaluating and reviewing all important processes.(For a discussion on how best to monitor and control health promotion work, see the section on "Evaluating the process" in Chapter 6.)

Obviously preventing problems is better than picking up problems after they have happened. Regularly reviewing and tightening up on all important specifications, reviewing the processes by which you implement the specifications, and developing and supervising your staff so that they take responsibility for quality, are taking the preventive approach further, and introducing systems for *"continuous quality improvement"*. In other words, once you have these systems in place, quality will be an integral part of everyone's work, not an additional extra. In practice, continuous quality improvement, quality assurance and quality control can be regarded as complementary (in the same way that health promotion, and diagnosis, treatment of illnesses, and rehabilitation and care, are complementary). What is important is the direction you are going in—towards managers taking on more of a facilitative (enabling) role and health promotion workers and teams taking increased control over their own work performance. Quality is thus as much about changing the way people relate to each other at work, and about making working life more satisfying, as it is about systems and standard setting.

QUALITY AND PARTICIPATION BY LOCAL PEOPLE IN HEALTH PROMOTION

Quality related to participation of local people in health promotion work involves a much more radical approach than simply assessing user satisfaction with what is provided. Health promotion seeks to share control of activities with the people concerned, which means involving them as much as possible in policy development, priority setting, planning and decision making about the style and range of health promotion programmes, projects and services.

Quality of participation related to health promotion provision thus starts with the *commissioning* process, and some health commissioners are testing new ways of gaining the active involvement of local people. In North Derbyshire, for example, *"The Safe Communities Project"* has targeted a local community with a high rate of accidents to children and recruited local people to train as interviewers of friends and neighbours in order to establish the causes of accidents and develop appropriate solutions (3). The solutions often turned out to be relatively inexpensive such as fencing off front gardens to prevent children from running onto the road and the provision of child safety equipment to less well off families.

At the provider level, local authorities, voluntary organizations and health service providers are increasingly encouraging active citizenship through employing community development workers or through training members of the community to act as community leaders. This is discussed further in Chapter 9.

Ideally, the views of local people should have equal weight alongside the views of professionals and other stakeholders, when making decisions about health promotion provisions. To take a very practical example of what this can mean, in many hospitals the tradition has been for patients to be prepared for sleep and awakening at times prescribed by the staff. Some hospitals are now allowing patients to go to sleep and wake up when they want. Patients prefer this, are more alert and active and eat better. The consequent disruption to ward routines has usually not been as difficult to manage as staff feared.

Another way of enabling more involvement by local people is through gathering information about their views and taking these into account when formulating policies and plans (i.e. through auditing the preferences and requirements of local people) (4). I discuss in detail what is meant by audit and how health promotion activities could be audited in the next chapter.

GETTING STARTED: GUIDELINES FOR PROVIDERS

The overall responsibility for a strategy for quality improvement must rest with managers. It will require time and effort from management before staff will be fully committed to quality improvement. I suggest, therefore, that the very first step for providers of health promotion might be to set up a quality improvement steering (coordinating) group, which has representation from managers in all the main functions of the business which are involved in the design and delivery of health promotion work. The role of this management group will be to develop a strategy for quality improvement, to coordinate the implementation of the strategy and to publicize and promote the strategy, so that the ground is thoroughly prepared, and anxieties of staff allayed, before any actual projects or initiatives are started. I suggest that the whole organization is alerted to the introduction of "quality improvement" as a permanent ongoing feature of the way to do health promotion work, with an explanation of the approach to be used.

I suggest a primarily "bottom-up" approach with the central coordinating/ steering group taking an enabling role, i.e. through delegating the actual development of systems to assure, control and continuously improve quality to the front-line practitioners and teams who do the health promotion work and to service users themselves. This way, staff and users will own the quality systems, and, of course, staff are the ones who are closest to the service users and who know what are critical areas from the users' point of view. They will also understand the system, because they have developed it themselves. Finally, the systems staff evolve in collaboration with service users are likely to be practical in the hurly-burly of the reality of working life. The people actually doing the health promotion work not only want to make a good job of it, but they usually are well aware of what is working and what isn't, and often know what is needed to put things right.

In the same way that managing for health gain involves completing the health gain cycle, improving quality involves completing a parallel quality cycle (see Figure 4.1). One way to get started is actually by intervening at

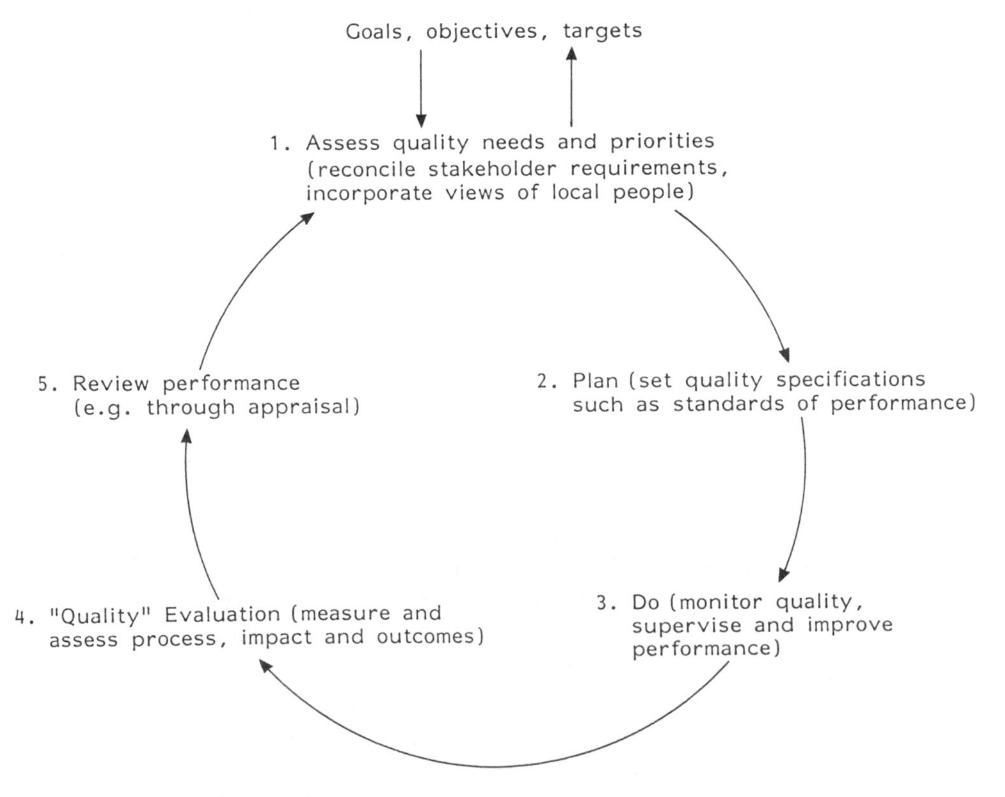

Figure 4.1 A quality cycle

the end of the cycle, and to start by reviewing (scrutinizing) some key quality features of current health promotion activities, or organizational processes, and thence identifying how performance can be improved, i.e. through the process of *audit*. (Audit is discussed in the next chapter.) Another way is through setting up one or more quality circles (i.e. quality action groups). Whichever way you start it should be the ideas of front-line staff and of the local people concerned which drive the engine of quality.

Quality circles

Quality circles are "action learning sets" (groups which meet regularly to help each other to improve the quality of work performance). Each quality action group focuses on improving the quality of the work of one particular function. They are one way of taking a bottom-up, staff-centred approach to quality improvement, and provide staff with opportunities for reflection, often alongside service users. Quality circles are "natural" work groups of between three and twelve employees (plus, perhaps, service users) who do the same or similar work (the term "circle" symbolizes the fact that all the members of the group are equally valuable). They meet voluntarily and regularly to support each other and find ways to improve quality. Service users are often invited to be members of quality circles, and may participate in activities such as quality improvement training. The aspects of quality they focus on are selected by the groups themselves and the outcomes are presented to management. Initially, managers may need to identify a suitable person (perhaps a staff development and training officer, or a health promotion specialist) to act as a facilitator of quality circles. Whoever the facilitator is, the important thing is that he or she is not a line manager of any of the staff involved. Quality circles are staff led, not management led. (The quality circle facilitators may need coaching or training on their role, for example in group work skills, such as how to adopt a people-centred, non-directive approach with quality circles, how to facilitate circles in identifying a range of options to improve quality, how to help groups to ensure confidentiality etc.) In time, through developing staff, facilitators will be drawn from within each staff group itself.

Quality circles work best where there are existing good relationships between managers and staff, and a sense of shared purpose. We have already discussed these preconditions in Chapter 2. It is also important to note that the solutions to problems and suggestions made by quality circles may have *costs*, and managers must be in a position to meet these when appropriate. If the suggestions made by quality circles, which have costs, are always rejected, staff will quickly lose commitment.

The questions members of quality circles could ask themselves, and gather information about, include:

- What are we trying to achieve (what is the purpose of our function related to health promotion)?
- How do we know when we are successful?
- How do others (e.g. our users) know when we are successful?
- What would top-quality health promotion work, in our situation, be like? (what is our vision of top-quality health promotion work?)
- What are the most important aspects of quality in health promotion to our stakeholders (all those with a vested interest in the outcomes) including purchasers, Trust Boards (e.g. chief executives, chairpersons and non-executive directors) and local people/patients/service users? (This may require some action research using techniques such as rapid appraisal, which I have already discussed in Chapter 3.) Different groups of stakeholders may have differing views on what are important aspects of quality, and it may be necessary to reconcile opposing views in order to establish priorities. The views of local people/patients/service users should be paramount.
- What quality improvements can we make to meet stakeholders'/local people's/patients' requirements more effectively and to move closer to our vision of top quality?
- How can we demonstrate that we are succeeding? (e.g. by setting, monitoring and reviewing standards, or by introducing systems for making regular checks on quality and continually improving quality, or by regularly reviewing our specifications and the processes by which they are implemented and met).

Typically, a quality circle will:

- Begin by drawing up a list of issues for consideration, using techniques such as brainstorming. (Brainstorming is a way of opening up a subject and collecting everyone's ideas without comment or criticisms.)
- Select the quality issue to be addressed.
- Gather, and analyse, information about the nature of the quality need.
- Generate a range of proposals to improve quality, and establish the best options or combination of options.
- Prepare a report on their processes, findings and recommendations, for decision by the quality management group.

For a case study on the health promotion work of a quality circle of nurses, see the note at the end of the chapter (5). For further reading on quality circles, see the suggestion in the note at the end of the chapter (6).

Quality circle members will often need training to carry their activities, such as training on how to identify key questions, on interviewing techniques (so that they avoid asking leading or ambiguous questions) and training in research methods such as questionnaire design and analysis. (For more about this, see the section on "Quality improvement training" later in this chapter.) For more information on how a quality circle might operate, see also the section on "How to conduct an audit" in Chapter 5. (The activities undertaken by quality circles and audit teams are similar, but they may start by intervening in the quality cycle at different points. Also, the focus of quality circles is narrower than an organizational audit, exploring how to improve the health promotion performance of just one particular function, such as occupational therapy, rather than scrutinizing the performance of all the functions in the organization involved.) See also the section on the skills of supervision, later in this chapter. The skills of peer appraisal are required by members of quality circles.

HOW TO SPECIFY THE QUALITY OF HEALTH PROMOTION WORK

Management systems need to ensure that quality is specified for a very wide range of items, including:

- Defining the health promotion orientation of the corporate mission of an organization, and health promotion policies, priorities, objectives and targets. (For a discussion of how to specify objectives and targets, see Chapter 6. For an example of a mission statement, see Chapter 3.)
- Describing the strategy for achieving health gain through health promotion activities. (For information related to specification of local health strategies, see Chapters 3 and 6.)
- Describing health promotion programmes, including defining expected outputs and outcomes and resource inputs, including staff training and standards of competence. (For a discussion of how to specify staff standards of competence, see Chapter 3.)
- Describing the accessibility and availability of programme components (such as projects and services); providing a clear description of what is to be provided by each component and what standards of performance, outputs and outcomes are expected; and describing the environments in which these are delivered.
- Describing the planning systems, including monitoring and evaluation procedures. (For a discussion on how to specify evaluation methods, see Chapter 6.)

Commissioners should primarily be concerned that quality management systems are in place, rather than the details of how the activities are provided. For example, it may be possible to achieve the outcomes through a number of different methods. Which methods to use, and the balance of different methods, should be left to providers, so that innovation is not stifled, and providers continue to experiment with finding the most effective methods for their circumstances.

However, commissioners may wish to specify key aspects of the policies they wish providers to pursue. So, for example, a health authority/health-commissioning agency might wish to specify what are the essential characteristics of organizations sponsoring health promotion activities. An example of such a specification by a health authority is set out in the following box.

Policy specification of a health authority related to sponsorship of health promotion activities

"Any organization sponsoring health promotion activities:

- Must not produce, promote or retail tobacco as a main product, nor be financially supported by tobacco companies.
- Must not promote the inappropriate use of alcohol.
- Must not produce or promote the consumption of foods which are detrimental to the health of people, whether in this country or overseas."

Quality standards

Standards are an important tool for specifying and assuring quality. Standards are agreed levels of performance negotiated within available resources. They are, however, only one part of a quality improvement system which aims for continually raising quality throughout all aspects of health promotion work. Standards are useful when you want to ensure consistency of key features of a service, and be able to compare quality across organizations, professional groups or geographical areas. However, standards do not necessarily assure (guarantee) high quality—they could be set too low, or so impossibly high that staff stop trying to reach them. Essentially, standards set a minimum which is attainable by everyone in a given set of circumstances. They are useful in four main areas of health promotion work:

- Related to *equity* in aspects such as access to health promotion provisions, and the design of services to meet special needs.

- Related to *user satisfaction* on issues such as provision of information, communication and quality of environments.
- Related to the *competence of professional staff* such as the standard of health education and health promotion performance by staff.
- Related to *quality of resources*, such as health information materials (for example, health promotion literature).

So, for example, standards could be set for health promotion leaflets, through identifying *criteria* to assess their quality, such as those set out in the following box.

Criteria for assessing the quality of health promotion leaflets (7)

- Appropriate for achieving your health promotion aims.
- Content consistent with your values and approach.
- Relevant for the people you are working with.
- Not racist or sexist.
- Easily understood by the people the leaflets are intended for.
- Contain accurate, up-to-date information.
- Free of inappropriate advertising.

A parent education course might set standards for:

- *User satisfaction*: for confirmation of places on a course (a possible standard might be within one week of referral or receiving applications).
- *Equity*: monitoring equity of access to courses (possible standards might be that clients living in deprived patches, or from disadvantaged or vulnerable groups, take up at least 50% of places on all courses; access is available for the disabled; a crèche is provided; affordable and convenient transport to the venue is available; the times are convenient for those wishing to attend).
- *Quality of resources*: monitoring quality of written and audiovisual material used on courses (standards could be that all written material has passed an appropriate readability test; all audiovisual material has been pre-tested with the target group; material is available in all the languages of those attending, and in Braille if required; subtitles ensure that audio material can be understood by people with hearing impairment).
- *Professional competence*: monitoring quality of the health education provided by staff (standards could be that the health education provided is based on an assessment of the needs of those attending, and

each session has a written plan including evaluation procedures; at the end of each course the impact on those attending is assessed and a review is conducted to identify ways of improving the course).

A further challenge is to develop standards which are *quantifiable* in some way. This is a difficult task, but you could, for example, develop a five-point scale for assessing the quality of your leaflets, so that you score them out of five for the extent to which they fulfil each quality criterion. Another example could be that you decide that a quality management issue is to respond quickly to requests from your clients. You could develop this by setting a standard such as returning telephone calls within 24 hours, and written requests within three days.

Setting, monitoring and reviewing standards can involve a great deal of time and effort. The benefit comes from seeing clearly identified improvements in service. Conversely, it is a waste of time to set standards and then neglect to monitor and review them regularly and use them to improve performance. The point of standards is that they can assist in improving performance. If they don't do this, staff will quickly get disillusioned with the whole process. Another problem with standards is that they are often reduced to a "paper-driven" exercise, when what is needed is quality monitoring and improvement through interpersonal discussions between practitioners and their peers, practitioners and users and between practitioners and managers. How to do this is discussed in the next section.

More information on specifying the quality of health promotion work can be found in the *Managing Health Improvement Project* (MAHIP) open learning materials (8). The development of national occupational standards (standards of professional competence) to provide quality benchmarks for health promotion work is discussed in Chapter 3. How to develop evaluation specifications is discussed in Chapter 6.

QUALITY MANAGEMENT OF PEOPLE

Supervision is an interpersonal process through which people are helped to improve work performance. It is a key aspect of managing *people* as opposed to managing money and material resources. Most of the money invested in health promotion is invested in people. The people management aspects of health promotion management are thus crucial. Yet the people management systems are often incomplete and fragmented. Good people management involves completing a people-orientated version of the basic quality cycle. It begins with setting and communicating business goals (defining the purpose of an organization) and then involves developing people to meet these goals through:

- Defining the purpose of each job, and thence the required goals, objectives, targets and standards of performance.
- Supervising performance through interpersonal discussions, focusing on congratulating successes and on identifying steps to be taken to improve performance when required.
- Implementing the development steps and thence the improvements.
- Review (appraisal: Have the targets and standards been reached? What do we need to do next?).

These stages are set out in cyclical form in Figure 4.2. The *Investors in People Standard* has been developed by the Employment Department nationally, to encourage employers to be effective in human resource development and to improve people's performance through setting and communicating business goals and developing people to meet these goals. The standard is

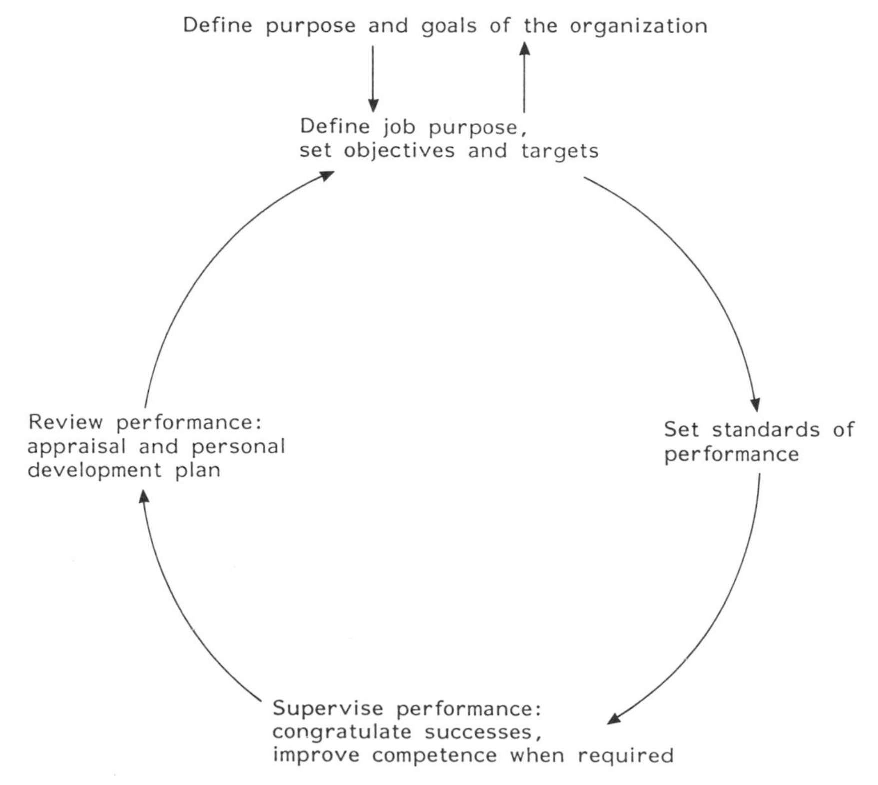

Figure 4.2 A people management cycle

based on national criteria and reflects good practice in training, development and organizational management, and hence gives assurances over the quality of the organization to employees, potential employees, customers and contractors (9).

Appraisal is a stock-take of the work performance of an individual (or a group of people), undertaken at an appropriate time in relation to their work activities (often on an annual basis), for the purpose of identifying what has happened during the previous period and what to do next (setting new objectives, improving standards of competence, etc.), including making a plan for the personal development of the individual or group concerned, in order to ensure that objectives and performance levels are achieved. Appraisal is thus the people management aspect of the review stage of the quality cycle. Appraisal and supervision are both needed to complete the people management cycle. Often, however, managers attempt to implement one part of the cycle without the other and the system then fails. For example, a manager insists on appraising staff whom he or she has failed to supervise. The manager then lacks insight into their work and their performance and is in no position to congratulate or to help and support further improvements. In fact the manager has not been there when needed and anything he or she says will have little credibility with the staff concerned.

There are some important reasons why managing people is often so badly handled. First, in our culture, we can have poor role models: parents and teachers and other powerful people in our childhood often ignore our achievements, and only comment when we do something wrong. We can be constantly judged for our mistakes but rarely praised for our successes. So, managers who behave like this are only copying what they have learned, it is not that they are "bad" people. Another reason is that in the past staff were often given the impression that once they were qualified, they were "kite-marked" as competent at their job for ever. So, if they fail to perform satisfactorily, they must be to blame! If they have training or development needs, this must be an admission of failure! Nowadays, in times of continual change, the nature of jobs is constantly changing, improved ways of working are constantly being discovered through research and the application of new technology, and constant learning and development are essential for everyone. Managers must therefore find new ways of relating to their staff, in order to reduce these barriers to high-quality work performance. The development of the skills required to be a good supervisor is a good place to start.

When supervision happens on a one-to-one basis, one person (the supervisor) helps another person (the supervisee) to improve his or her work performance. *Managerial supervision* happens when the supervisor is also the line manager of the supervisee. Managerial supervision provides the quality control over the work of staff, through ensuring that the standards of the agency in which the work is being done are upheld and through identifying ways of improving performance. Supervision should not be limited to helping *individuals* to monitor and learn from their own performance. *Teams, departments* and *whole organizations* need to be supervised in order to learn and develop from their experience. It is important, therefore, for all organizations, departments and directorates etc. to have policies on supervision and appraisal (i.e. on how to manage people), which clearly state:

- *Why* supervision and appraisal are important (to ensure quality of work performance; to improve staff motivation and morale; to ensure quality is continually improved; to improve teamwork; to develop the whole organization).
- *Who* should receive supervision and appraisal from *whom* (for example, staff from line managers, trainees from supervisors, professionals from more senior professionals, teams from team leaders and each other, whole organizations from their executive board, peers from each other). Mechanisms are needed for *upward* appraisal (appraisal of senior managers and directors by more junior staff; appraisal of staff by service users), as well as top-down and sideways appraisal (co-appraisal by peers).
- *When* and how frequently each should happen.
- *How* they should be carried out—what sort of approach (a developmental one rather than a judgemental one). Supervision and appraisal should be empowering processes, liberating staff to develop their skills to "do things better", and to enhance their contribution to the organization ("do better things").
- *What* they should focus on—personal and organizational development.
- *How* training will be provided for all concerned. Enhanced communication skills are essential.

The next section focuses on the communication skills required by a manager to implement continuous quality improvement in health promotion work through *one specific approach to supervision* of staff. It is based on a model first developed by Steve de Shazer (10) at the Brief Family Therapy Centre in Milwaukee, and later used with clients with a range of difficulties at the Marlborough Family Service, Bloomsbury Health Authority and the Parkside Clinic, Parkside Health Authority (11). It is essentially a brief and effective approach to mutual empowerment, which I have adapted for use by managers seeking to empower staff to take responsibility for their own work performance (i.e., it is a method of *value-adding* supervision).

Although I focus here on the use of the approach by managers when supervising staff, this could, of course, be used in other contexts, for example:

- To *provide a role model for staff to adopt with others*, for example to empower their own staff, or to empower clients wishing to change their lifestyles (see Chapter 9 for more about this).
- During *professional supervision* (supervision of a professional by a more experienced and competent member of the profession).
- During *mentoring* (mentoring is the process by which a more experienced manager or professional—a *mentor*—assists a *mentee* to improve his or her work performance. The mentor acts as an unbiased coach and guide, and is not the line manager of the mentee).
- As an approach to *staff appraisal* (an in-depth review of the performance of a member of staff, usually undertaken by the member of staff and his or her manager, in order to establish how the person can best be helped to further improve performance and to formulate a personal development plan).
- As a method of *team development* through peer supervision and appraisal (this is discussed briefly at the end of the section).

Its disadvantage could be that through focusing on *continuously improving* performance, it could fail to address how to deal with *extremely poor* performance. It is therefore only one approach to supervision, which complements others, and you must use your judgement (and the guidance provided by your organization's policy) about when it is appropriate. It is necessary to face the reality that, however skilled you are, it may not be possible to improve the performance of some individuals. For further reading on the principles and practice of supervision, a detailed consideration of which is beyond the scope of this book, see the suggestions in the note at the end of this chapter (12).

The skills of value-adding supervision

The value-adding model of supervision described here is based on two assumptions:

1. Knowing about the problems or current situation experienced by a person is less useful than helping the individual to construct a view of the desired future (what would top-quality health promotion work be like in my situation?).
2. Focus on what the person is already doing to move towards that outcome.

The approach thus focuses on building the confidence of a person that he or she has the capacity to change, through encouraging a focus on *successes* (what the person is already doing to reach the outcome), rather than focusing on past mistakes or failures. The manager using this approach is acting as a change agent through encouraging the person to identify and use their own strengths, qualities and resources and to continually move towards the desired outcome. The manager does this through guiding the discussions towards a clearer vision of the outcome.

This may involve examining different viewpoints on the outcome:

1. The views of the member of staff.
2. The views of the manager.
3. The views of the users.
4. The views of the organization.
5. The views of other key people with an interest in the outcome.

The more nearly these coincide, the more likely is success. Where these do not match, the manager may be able to facilitate better congruence, for example through redesigning the job of the staff member, or perhaps through enabling the employee to shadow a more highly experienced professional (13).

Because the manager actively directs the conversation towards outcomes, this could be construed as an authoritarian approach. This is a misconception, since it is vital that the manager neither tells the person how to change, nor imposes his or her views. Using this approach elicits a person's own way of doing things, rather than making them a clone of the manager. It is thus about power sharing and enabling people to take power. The manager guides the conversation by the choice of particular questions and the language used to frame them. Practice in the development and use of appropriate questions is important for skill development. The questions focus on the here-and-now or the future (and only touch on the past when looking for past successes). Questions are essentially of two types:

1. Reporting questions: questions which ask the employee to report on thoughts, actions and feelings, related to successes. For example:
   - What has been helpful to you so far in our discussions?
   - How do you account for that?
2. Change-orientated questions: probing questions which help to construct a vision of the changes required to move towards the outcome, through probing specific aspects of change, or through comparing and contrasting the desired future with the present situation. For example:
   - What would the result be if you were successful?
   - What would be your criteria for success?

- What indicators would show success?
- How will you know that the staff team are performing better?
- What will be different when relationships with the local authority are improved?
- What will you need to see that will tell you that you are on track (or tell you that this work has succeeded)?
- What will you be doing that will be different when you have made this change?

It is essential for the manager to phrase these questions carefully. For example, to say: "What changes have happened since I last saw you?" rather than "Have any changes happened ...?" Questions that can be answered with a "yes" or "no" are best avoided. Use language which helps the employee to see a picture of concrete, specific changes. Don't ask the person "What do you need to do differently?" This is too vague. Ask him or her to picture the goals or desired results, and the steps towards this will begin to come clearer. The more a detailed picture of the outcome is built up, the clearer will be the range of possibilities for actions to reach it.

Other useful questions to ask are:

"What do *I* have to do differently to make this meeting work for you?"

"What, if anything, in this meeting has been useful to you?" "What has it changed?"

The stages of value-adding supervision: the first session (goal setting)

The purpose of the first session is to establish goals and to begin movement towards them. This is done through "change talk" which focuses on the member of staff determining his or her own goals, and scanning for examples of what the employee already does which is useful towards attaining the goals. The employee is then encouraged to find more ways of using these strengths in a wider range of situations or contexts. The employee is encouraged to picture what it will be like at work when the goals have been reached. This positive picture becomes the overall goal and serves as a yardstick by which progress can be measured. The discussion clarifies further what it will be like at work when the goals are reached, thus conveying to the employee that the changes are not only possible but realistically achievable. Feedback from the manager is positive only, complimenting the employee on achievements.

The final part of the first session is concerned with task setting (setting tasks to be carried out before the next interview). The nature of these interventions will depend on the "position" of the employee. At this stage, employees can be described in terms of three categories:

1. *Unmotivated*: an employee who does not want to discuss his or her work performance with the manager and who is resisting change.
2. *Undecided*: these employees are unsure whether talking to the boss will help but recognize that changes are needed to improve services or programmes.
3. *Motivated*: these employees want to provide quality services and welcome help with how to do it.

Unmotivated employees may be pessimistic about improving quality and interested only in "getting managers off their backs". In these cases the focus of the interview would be on how this could be achieved, and on giving complimentary feedback only (no tasks would be set). Sometimes unmotivated staff will be sufficiently influenced by the manager's view of their capacity for change to move into another category. The experiences of other staff may also influence an employee to move, at a later date, from "unmotivated" to "undecided" or to "motivated".

"Undecideds" may be given observation tasks, such as "Notice what is different about the times when you meet with your team", "Observe what is happening at work that you want to continue."

"Doing tasks" are reserved for motivated staff who are eager to change and hope that the session will help them to achieve change. The employee may be simply asked to do those things which have been defined as "successes" in the interview and to notice "what you are doing when there are more changes". Or the employee may be set a more specific task, such as a "rating" task. This involves asking employees where on a scale from 0 (worst performance) to 10 (best performance) they think they are at in terms of standards of work performance related to a key results area. The manager can then ask "What would you settle for as a realistic standard in the circumstances?" This then defines the goal. If, for example, an employee rates her performance as a 3, and a realistic standard as a 7, the manager then asks her to notice what she is doing when she's at 4, 5 or 6. Thus the task is noticing improved performance. Through noticing what is happening when performance is improved, the employee begins to identify what are the steps needed to improve performance.

Subsequent sessions (assessing change over time)

The purpose of each subsequent session is to assess change and to help to maintain it so that goals can be achieved. The manager starts the next session where he or she left off. So, if the task was to notice something, start by asking what the employee has noticed. Or the manager could ask "What have you been doing that's been good for your work performance?" If goal-directed behaviour is described, build on this as much as possible with lots of compliments and "change talk". Use the whole range of questions, described in the first session, to explore what needs to happen for the desired behaviour to happen again and more often. The main thing is to communicate to staff your belief in *their own* ability to change things—that it's under their control, not yours.

If staff report no change or even that things are worse, do not initially accept this at face value. For example, precisely because the employee's expectations of what can be achieved has been raised, they may be less tolerant of things they were previously able to tolerate. Or the employee may not have appreciated the significance of changes, and thus fails to report them as positive change. So thoroughly explore any differences in what is happening and use "change talk" to identify the changes.

If things really have not improved, explore any possible explanations for lack of change. Asking what the member of staff is doing to prevent matters from getting worse can yield useful information regarding his or her strengths. It could be that the goals were unrealistic in the circumstances, and that more realistic goals need to be identified.

Team development through peer supervision and appraisal

The approach described above can also be used by teams responsible for the achievement of shared objectives (for example, a quality circle), or by the staff of a department or directorate responsible for delivery of specific programmes or services (for example, the administrative staff), as a method of peer supervision and support and peer appraisal. In this context it concentrates on identifying the goals of the team, or function, and the steps which can be taken to reach those goals, through:

- Using the strengths, qualities and resources of the team/staff.
- Identifying successes (what the team/group of staff is already doing which helps movement towards the goals).
- Giving each other only positive feedback.
- Using "change talk" to improve performance.

It follows that peer supervision is a tool for not only identifying current standards of performance of a group of people, but also for continuously raising standards, through a team or group of staff setting, reviewing and improving their own standards. (For further discussion of team development, see Chapter 7.)

As with one-to-one supervision, this approach will complement the formal staff appraisal system (individual performance review), which is set out in the policies of the organization. If the staff appraisal system authorized by management does not command the respect and commitment of staff, then it may be difficult to introduce additional ways of assessing staff performance and of learning and developing. Managerial supervision and peer supervision flourish best in a "learning culture" and a "learning organization". It is vital for managers, therefore, to demonstrate to staff that they are not experts in everything, and are actively learning themselves! It may also be necessary for you to use your influence to improve the staff appraisal and supervision policies of your organization (14).

THE ROLE OF THE MANAGER IN PROFESSIONAL DEVELOPMENT

There are a large number of different ways of developing professionals and thence spreading good practice, such as networking, journal clubs (clubs where members take turns to read journals and report on what they have learnt to colleagues) and coaching, and I do not attempt to cover all of them here (15). I focus on how the manager can play a key role in encouraging good practice.

A research-based approach

First you must know what works and what is ineffective. This means that practice must be based on a firm foundation of research and development (R&D) (16). Knowledge and understanding of what is good practice must be gathered. Professional bodies such as the British Dietetic Association, the Institution of Environmental Health Officers, the Royal College of Nursing, and the Health Visitors Association, to name but a few, have an important role here, in the dissemination of good practice, as have institutions of higher education and training, so that staff are developed and competent to perform their roles. (I have already discussed education, training and staff development in more detail in Chapter 3.) Managers must ensure that the work of their service is research based, and that staff are continuously developed in order to deliver "current best practice" in their health promotion work. The guidelines used by staff should have the following characteristics (17):

1. They are informed by formal systematic literature reviews of the research evidence.
2. Recommendations should be firmly based on evidence of effectiveness and cost-effectiveness.
3. Purchasers and providers agree criteria for the review of practice based on guidelines, and a schedule for the regular review of guidelines.

Without these safeguards guidelines can simply be a mechanism for managers or others to impose their preferred approach to practice on front-line staff.

Encouraging professional quality

> The most valuable things in the (public) service are the professionalism and commitment of staff, which have been eroded and need to be nurtured. Quality reverses the downward spiral. A quality approach can be introduced in a way that connects with staff values and concerns and offers a realistic and worth-while way forward.
>
> But quality methods should not be presented only as a way of defending a service, or as something which resonates with and advances core values. It also has to be shown to provide something tangible for staff, as something that will help them to protect their jobs and acquire necessary skills in competitive markets. As something which will save time in the long run and remove the headaches and common complaints at work.
>
> John Øvretveit (18)

It is vital that managers work together with professionals to identify ways of improving quality which make work less frustrating, give the professionals more control, and defuse user dissatisfaction by negotiating expectations. It is important, therefore, for managers to regularly review and improve arrangements for maintaining staff commitment, knowledge, motivation and competence related to the health promotion aspects of their work. Factors which should improve motivation include good quality supervision and performance appraisal systems which command the respect and commitment of staff (for example, through using the approach to peer supervision discussed in the previous section, in addition to individual performance review), training, and autonomous working teams.

Facilitation

You can play a direct role in spreading good health promotion practice by facilitating professional quality, through supervising your professional staff, or through encouraging team development (as previously described), or through arranging for and supporting supervision of staff by more experienced and competent professionals—*professional supervision*. You can also encourage and legitimize mechanisms for *peer* supervision, for example, through pairs, or small groups of staff, who have the same or similar roles, meeting regularly to explore how to improve performance.

You could encourage professions to develop mechanisms for regular *upward appraisal*.

Quality improvement training

Training in the principles and skills of quality improvement is an essential component of any quality improvement strategy. The training must give participants a structured overview of the quality improvement process (for example, through using the cyclical model described in this chapter) and provide them with skills training. With respect to quality improvement, the training itself must, of course, be of high quality and there are at least three levels to which quality judgements can be applied:

- The quality of the training itself.
- The quality of the work activity of those trained (the steps staff take to improve quality).
- The quality of the outputs and outcomes of the activities of those trained (whether quality is actually improved).

Quality improvement training specifically related to health promotion is in its infancy. I suggest that it might be designed using the following principles:

Principles for health promotion quality improvement training

- Training should be multidisciplinary and suitable for all health promoters whether they work in health, education, social services, voluntary organizations, environmental health, commercial businesses and workplaces or other settings.
- Training should cover both the theory and practice of quality improvement and audit relevant to health promotion work and should give participants the opportunity to practise the skills they are taught.
- Training should be designed to meet the specific needs of those attending. It should therefore be preceded by a needs assessment process, conducted in collaboration with senior managers and health promotion workers from interested local agencies and businesses. The goals and

continued on next page

continued

objectives of the training should be agreed by all participating organizations.

- The training should be structured round a health gain cycle and a quality improvement cycle, such as Figure 1.1 and Figures 4.1, 4.2 and 4.3 in this book, with participants using these cycles to organize their own quality improvement and health promotion work.
- Training should be linked to workplace quality activities, such as workplace action learning sets, team development, audit projects and research.
- Training should be evaluated at three levels: the training itself, the work activity of those trained, and the outcomes of the training. Evaluation methods and procedures should be agreed by all participating organizations before the training starts, and should be a shared, collaborative process.
- Training materials should be flexible so that they can be adjusted to meet the needs of different staff groups and take account of feedback from participants as each course goes along.
- The training should be so designed that a wide variety of facilitators, from different backgrounds, can run the courses, thus using training expertise from the range of participating organizations.
- The aim should be that the training, and its outputs and outcomes, are "owned" by all the participating organizations.

Training in health promotion work

In health promotion work the ultimate outcome desired is the improved health of local people and communities. This is achieved by the improvement in the quality of the health promotion work of the professionals trained. It is thus essential that professionals are aware of the current standards of their health promotion practice, and of what is best practice, and that training is designed specifically to improve the professional health promotion performance of those trained. Recent publications in *The Health of the Nation* series address the issues of defining good practice for some of the key professions involved in health promotion work (19).

Identifying the health promotion role

One of the reasons why spreading good practice in health promotion can be neglected is that professionals fail to identify the health promotion aspects of their work and to discriminate between their health promotion work and their specialist work, such as enforcing legislation (in the work of environmental health officers) or treating a wound (in the work of nurses) or providing care (in the work of carers). Guidance on how to identify health promotion work is provided in Chapter 3, and in more detail in Ewles and Simnett (20).

Evaluation

Finally, evaluation is an essential element of good professional practice. All activities, however modest, should be evaluated, and professionals should be encouraged to share the findings of their evaluations, both within and across professions. (Evaluation is discussed in more detail in Chapter 6.)

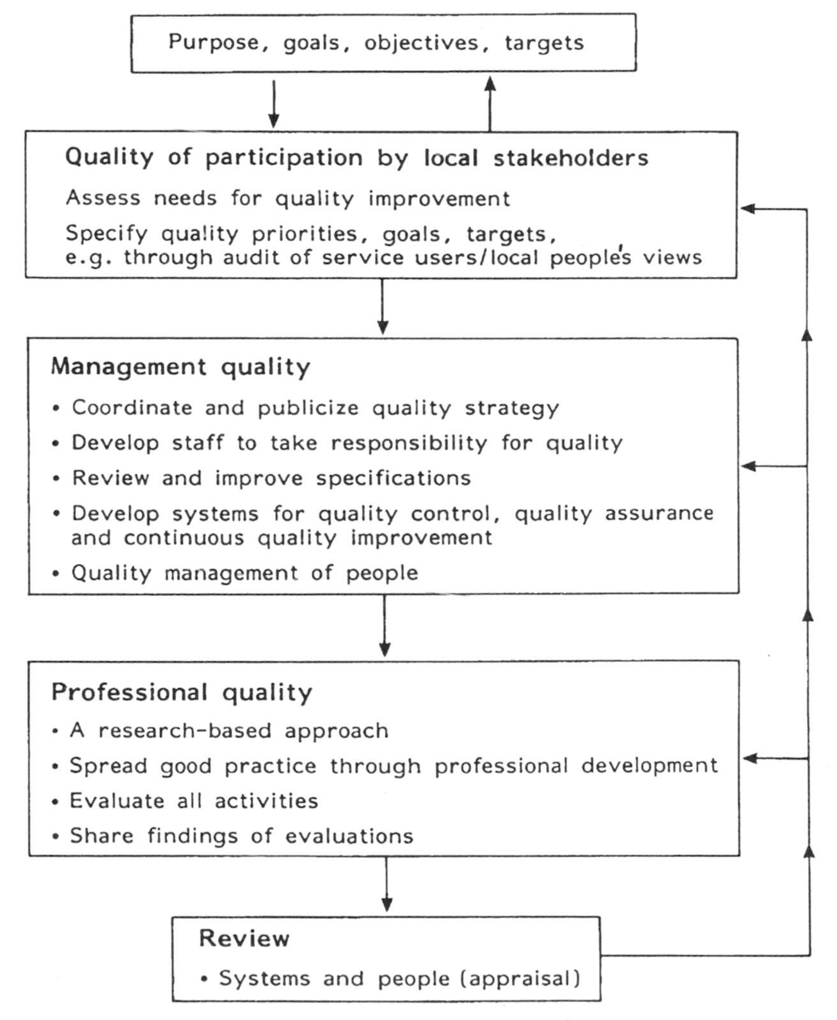

Figure 4.3 The key elements of a quality improvement system for health promotion work

Managers need systems to monitor and review all these aspects of professional performance in order to control the quality of health promotion practice.

There is considerable literature on improving quality, and suggestions for further study are given (21). The key elements of a quality improvement system for health promotion work are summarized in Figure 4.3. Note that this is actually a quality-focused version of the "health gain spiral" which I introduced in Chapter 1. Thus, continuous quality improvement systems build in quality at every stage of the health gain spiral: stage 1—assess needs; stage 2—plan; stage 3—do; stage 4—evaluate; and stage 5—review. Achieving health gain can thus be conceptualized as involving a multilayered process, with a quality cycle and a people management cycle superimposed on the basic planning–doing–evaluating–reviewing health gain cycle.

In summary, *quality* is:

> a continuous, never-ending commitment to improvement.

Introducing a quality improvement system is a developmental process. It is about the gradual introduction of quality ideas and methods into the work of an organization or department or team, through using the ideas of the staff and of service users. Start with something small and specific. It could be that auditing one aspect of your work will be the catalyst for development. This is what I turn to in the next chapter.

An activity you could undertake

- Working in groups of three colleagues, take turns to talk about a key results area in which you want to improve your performance. One of your colleagues should interview you, using the skills of peer supervision, previously discussed. The second colleague should act as an active observer, making suggestions to the interviewer about how to improve the questions and guide the discussions, both during the interview and afterwards.
- Then share your feelings and thoughts about this approach to peer supervision. How is it different from previous experiences you have had? Are the results different?

Questions you could ask yourself

- What forces are helping me to improve the quality of health promotion work? (Think of people, relationships, resources, organizational issues, environment, etc.)

continued on next page

continued

- What forces are hindering me from improving the quality of health promotion work?
- What could I do to increase the helping forces and decrease the hindering forces? (Reducing the resistance is likely to be the most powerful intervention, rather than pushing harder.)

NOTES, REFERENCES AND FURTHER READING

(1) I outline here how some of the key terms, used in discussions on quality of health promotion work, which are used in this book:

Quality in health promotion: "Meeting the requirements of those who most need help to prevent illness and improve health, at the lowest cost and within policies set by higher authorities." This definition is taken from the paper by Dr John Øvretveit "Improving the quality and effectiveness of health promotion programmes," presented at a conference on Health Promotion Quality, held on 14 February 1994 and hosted by the Health Development Team of the London Borough of Richmond. For further information about this conference and its report, see note (19).

Standard: an agreed level of performance achievable within available resources.

Audit: there is no general agreement about the meaning of this term. In this book I use it to mean a critical scrutiny of important parts of an organization, alliance, policy, programme, project or service, followed by the implementation of recommendations to improve quality. Audit can either involve an internal review carried out by those responsible for providing or managing an organization or activity (see *Review*), or scrutiny by an independent external auditor, such as the Audit Commission. Audit can also be consumer-led through gathering and acting on local people's views. Audit is a systematic process for improving service quality and outcomes through comparing what is done with agreed best practice (e.g., nationally agreed standards) and identifying ways of delivering best practice, and/or through identifying and resolving quality problems in the process of service delivery.

Review: the critical analysis of specific components of health promotion work, conducted by those responsible for carrying out and/or managing the work, or by consumers (local people), or by external assessors, at an appropriate point in time, in order to reflect on what has happened, how it could be improved and what to do next. Review is an essential stage in the quality cycle. It is a process of "taking stock" at one particular point in time.

Appraisal: a cooperative process of staff members' appraising their own development, their own strengths and weaknesses and then receiving feedback on and refinement of their own self-appraisals from their peers and/or their manager. A good appraisal system focuses not just on performance, but also on what staff members have learnt, how they have developed and how their learning and development can best take place and be nurtured in the future. It forms the "review" stage of the managing people cycle.

Monitoring: continuous or regularly repeated observations or checks on important parts of an input, process, output or outcome.

Inputs: all the resources that go into activities, including staffing, money, materials and time.

Process: what happens between inputs and outcomes.

Outputs: the results of an activity in terms of the provision of facilities, services or procedures implemented, for example the services and facilities available to patients of a GP.

Outcomes: the achievement or end-product of an activity, expressed in appropriate terms, such as changes in people's attitudes, knowledge or behaviour, changes in health policy, changes in the uptake of preventive services, or health gain, as measured by health outcome indicators.

Impact: in this book I use the term to mean all the consequences that can be attributed to an activity, such as changes in the activities of other people, changes in processes and procedures, provision of services and facilities, environmental change and organizational change. The impact includes the intended results (outputs and outcomes) of an activity, and also any unintended consequences. The term is sometimes used specifically to describe short-term outcomes. For example, the *impact* of a programme to encourage women to attend for a breast-screening test (mammography) might be assessed in terms of how many women attended: the long-term *outcome* would be a change in the rate of women who died of breast cancer.

Quality assurance: an approach which aims to prevent poor quality by setting standards.

Quality control: a system for inspecting things and identifying items which do not meet standards.

Continuous quality improvement: a system which goes further than quality assurance because it puts emphasis on each employee owning responsibility for quality and its improvement. The manager's role becomes one of facilitating the achievement of high quality by employees. Continuous quality improvement thus enables employees to improve the quality of health promotion work through increasing their control over their own performance. Quality becomes an integral part of all activities rather than an add-on extra.

Cost effectiveness: establishing the cost and effectiveness of an activity in relation to a desired outcome. This could be through determining which of a number of alternative activities require the lowest cost input for a given outcome, or through determining which activity will produce the highest effectiveness for a given cost input. In health promotion work, outcome measures could include health gain, or changes in behaviour which may be expected to lead to health gain, such as reducing the numbers of people who smoke, or changes in environmental conditions which may be expected to lead to health gain, such as reducing levels of air pollution.

Effectiveness: the extent to which an activity provides benefit for an individual or a community.

Efficiency: the relationship between the inputs and outputs of an activity. An efficient activity is one that maximizes the outputs for a given input, or *minimizes* input for a fixed output.

Specification: the document that describes in detail the requirements with which a resource, policy, activity or service has to comply.

(2) Øvretveit, J. (1992) *Health Service Quality*. Oxford: Blackwell Scientific Publications.

(3) Layzell, A. (1994) Local and vocal: perspectives on purchasing. *Health Service Journal* **104** (5386): 28–29.

(4) How to audit the views of health service users is discussed in: Bradburn, J. (1994) Eye opener: consumer audit. *Health Service Journal* **104** (5414): 20–21.

(5) See:

Ewles, L. and Simnett, I. (3rd edn, 1995) *Promoting Health: A Practical Guide*. London: Scutari Press. Ch. 7.

(6) Transport and General Workers Union (1989) *Employee Involvement and Quality Circles*. London: TGWU.

(7) These criteria are based on criteria identified in:

Ewles, L. and Simnett, I. (3rd edn, 1995) *Promoting Health: A Practical Guide*. London: Scutari Press. Ch. 7.

(8) The *Managing Health Improvement Project* (MAHIP) volume entitled *Quality Issues in Health Promotion Work*, which was written by Ina Simnett, Pat Dark, Moira Bremner, and Pat Evans, focuses on quality.

For further information about the availability of these materials, see note (8) in Chapter 1.

(9) For further information about *Investors in People* (IIP), see the booklet: *Invest in Success* (1992), available from the Employment Department, Moorfoot, Sheffield S1 3PQ.

To find out more about how your organization could gain recognition, contact your local Training and Enterprise Council (TEC).

The NHS Training Division is taking a leading role in highlighting the value of *Investors in People* in the NHS, through a programme of regional workshops. For information about these, contact the NHS Training Division (NHSTD), St Bartholomews Court, 18 Christmas Street, Bristol BS1 5BT. Telephone: 0117 9291029.

(10) De Shazer, S. (1985) *Keys to Solution in Brief Therapy*, New York: Norton.

(11) Evan, G., Iveson, C. and Ratner, H. (1990) *Problem to Solution: Brief Therapy with Individuals and Families*. London: Brief Therapy Press. Available from: Brief Therapy Press, 17 Avenue Mansions, Finchley Road, London NW3 7AX. Telephone: 0171 794 4495.

Brief Therapy Practice provides training in the skills of brief therapy for workers from health, social services and education, and for supervisors. Further information is available from: Brief Therapy Practice, 77 Muswell Avenue, London N10 2EH. Telephone: 0181 883 6848.

(12) You may have a negative concept of supervision, based on your own experiences of it. Gaie Houston provides a definition of the sort of supervision I am referring to, in the Foreword to her book on supervision:

"I asked a young therapist who comes to me for supervision what she expected from our sessions. She said 'You know, a sort of looking at the whole thing in perspective. I want really *super* vision.' She was not primarily asking that I should have this god-like overview. She wanted it for herself, as a product of what went on between us."

Houston. G. (1990) *Supervision and Counselling*. London: Rochester Foundation.

One solution to negative perceptions of supervision can be to rename it as "consultation".

Two audio tapes providing training in supervision have been produced by Franceska Inskipp and Brigid Proctor: "Skills for Supervisees" and "Skills for Supervisors". These are available from Alexia Publications, c/o Brigid Proctor, 4 Ducks Walk, Twickenham, Middlesex.

A good introduction to the principles and practice of supervision in the helping professions is provided in:

Hawkins, P. and Shohet, R. (1989) *Supervision in the Helping Professions: An Individual, Group and Organisational Approach.* Milton Keynes: Open University Press.

General texts are:

Evans, D. (1991) *Supervisory Management: Principles and Practice.* London: Cassell Educational.

Irwin, R. and Wolenik, R. (1986) *Winning Strategies for Managing People: A Task Directed Guide.* London: Kogan Page.

(13) *Shadowing* provides an opportunity for one individual to experience and understand the role and work practices of another in order to improve performance, develop the organization, or to explore career opportunities. For more information on shadowing see:

NHS Executive (1994) *Shadowing: Management Development for NHS Staff.* London: Department of Health.

This booklet can be obtained from the Health Publications Unit: BAPS, Health Publications Unit, Heywood Stores, No. 2 Site, Manchester Road, Heywood, Lancs OL10 2PZ.

(14) *Networking* is about getting to know people other than your immediate colleagues, who are working in the same field, and using the information

you share to improve performance. For further information on networking, see:

NHS Executive (1994) *Networking: A Guide for Nurses, Midwives, Health Visitors and the Professions Allied to Medicine.* London: Department of Health.

This booklet can be obtained from the Health Publications Unit; see the address under note (13).

(15) For help with constructing an effective appraisal system, see:

Hudson, H. (1992) *The Perfect Appraisal: All You Need to Get it Right First Time.* London: Century Business.

(16) For information about the evidence for identifying some health promotion methods as being more effective for particular aims, see:

Tones, K. and Tilford, S. (2nd edn, 1994) *Health Education: Effectiveness, Efficiency and Equity.* London: Chapman & Hall.

Bunton, R. and Macdonald, G. (eds) (1992) *Health Promotion: Disciplines and Diversity.* London: Routledge.

(17) Much of the guidance on valid clinical practice guidelines in the following article can equally apply to health promotion practice guidelines:

Sheldon, T., Freemantle, N., Grimshaw, J. and Russell, I. (1994) The guide to good guides. *Health Service Journal* **104** (5432): 34–35.

See also:

Bulletin No. 8 (1994) *Effective Health Care: Implementing Clinical Guidelines.* Leeds: Leeds University.

Available from: Effective Health Care, Nuffield Institute for Health, 71 Clarendon Road, Leeds LS2 9PL. Telephone: 01904 433668.

(18) Øvretveit, J. (1992) *Therapy Services: Organisation, Management and Autonomy.* Chur, Switzerland: Harwood Academic Publishers.

(19) The *Health of the Nation* publications currently available on good practice are:

Department of Health (1993) *Targeting Practice: The Contribution of Nurses, Midwives and Health Visitors.*

Institution of Environmental Health Officers (1993) *The Health of the Nation for Environmental Health.*

Department of Health (1994) *Targeting Practice: The Contribution of State Registered Dieticians.*

These documents, with the exception of the one on environmental health, can be obtained from the Health Publications Unit; see the address under note (13). *The Health of the Nation for Environmental Health* can be obtained from The Institution of Environmental Health Officers, Chadwick Court, 15 Hatfields, London, SE1 8DJ. Telephone: 0171 928 6006.

(20) A map of all the activities subsumed in health promotion work, and a detailed description of the core competencies required for health promotion work, can be found in:

Ewles, L. and Simnett, I. (3rd edn, 1995) *Promoting Health: A Practical Guide*. London: Scutari Press. Ch. 2.

(For an explanation of what is meant by "core competencies", see the discussion on training in Chapter 3.)

(21) For a useful quality assurance framework for health promotion, and examples of quality standards, see:

Evans, D., Head, M.J. and Speller, V. (1994) *Assuring Quality in Health Promotion: Developing Standards of Good Practice*. London: Health Education Authority.

The report of a conference on Quality in Health Promotion, supported by the Society of Health Education and Health Promotion Specialists, and hosted by the Health Development Team, London Borough of Richmond upon Thames on 14 February 1994, contains three very useful papers. Copies of this report can be obtained from:

Health Development Officer, 1st Floor, Civic Centre, 44 York Street, Twickenham TW1 3BZ Telephone: 0181 891 7488.

For textbooks on quality related to health care, see:

Wright, C. and Whittington, D. (1992) *Quality Assurance: An Introduction for Health Care Professionals*. Edinburgh: Churchill Livingstone.

Ellis, R. and Whittington, D. (1993) *Quality Assurance in Health Care: A Handbook*. London: Edward Arnold.

Øvretveit, J. (1992) *Health Service Quality*. Oxford: Blackwell Scientific Publications.

Øvretveit, J. (1994) *Purchasing for Health*. Milton Keynes: Open University Press.

For a text on the use of continuous quality improvement methods in health care settings in the USA, see:

Berwick, D., Godfrey, A. and Rossener, J. (1990) *Curing Healthcare: New Strategies for Quality Improvement*. San Francisco: Jossey Bass.

For a general (UK) text on continuous quality improvement, see:

Pike, J. and Barnes, R. (1994) *TQM in Action: A Practical Approach to Continuous Performance Improvement*. London: Chapman & Hall.

For a critique of current approaches to quality improvement in the NHS, see:

Øvretveit, J. (1994) TQM has failed in the NHS. *Health Service Journal* **104** (5341): 24–26.

CHAPTER 5 Audit and the management of health promotion

Summary

This chapter discusses some key issues related to audit of health promotion. It starts by discussing what it is and clarifies this through comparing audit with other related activities (research and evaluation). It continues by discussing why audit is necessary; how it could be tackled in a systematic but comprehensive way across all the diverse agencies concerned; what methods might be used; who could do it in a manner which will ensure high-quality audits; what criteria could be used to decide when an audit is needed; and how to ensure accountability to all those with an interest in the outcomes of health promotion work. It includes a case study on auditing health promotion activity, and ends with some questions you could ask yourself.

WHAT IS AUDIT?

Audit is the process of scrutinizing the operations of an organization, alliance, department, service, project, policy or programme, for the purpose of improving performance and ensuring accountability. Its ultimate purpose is to improve quality and outcomes, and to ensure that activities meet the requirements of local people. It is, perhaps, best viewed as a systematic *method* for improving quality and/or for ensuring that health promotion meets the needs of local people. It therefore contributes to the quality cycle and to quality improvement systems. It can involve carrying out an in-depth internal review (part of "self-audit" or "peer audit") by those responsible for providing or managing health promotion, or an external scrutiny by independent *auditors*. Whoever conducts the audit, it is a process of taking stock of the management of health promotion activities, or of the management of health-promoting organizations/alliances, conducted at appropriate points in the lifetime of activities or of the organization/alliance, and of implementing measures to improve quality.

The *output* of an audit is a report (or perhaps several reports) which make recommendations about how to improve systems, processes and ways of working. The *outcome* of audit is that recommendations are implemented and quality is improved.

The differences between audit, research and evaluation

It is difficult to discriminate between audit and other similar activities, so it can help to clarify matters by highlighting the differences and similarities. These are set out in the following box.

Comparing research, audit and evaluation

Research

Both research and audit involve the collection and examination of data, but the purpose is different. Research is concerned with generating *new knowledge and new approaches which have general application.* Audit is concerned with what works, or doesn't work, in particular local circumstances. Research may be concerned with *efficacy* (whether an intervention actually works). Audit is concerned with *effectiveness* (whether an intervention, which has been shown to work, does so in practice in particular local circumstances), and *efficiency* (whether resources are being used to the best advantage by a particular department or team). So the findings of an audit relate to the work of a particular team, organization or alliance, or to delivering a particular programme, in specific local circumstances.

Audit

Audit is concerned with management systems and processes: the performance of organizations and alliances, the quality of their services and outputs and the accountability of public sector organizations for the funds which are allocated to them. Audit, therefore, looks at activities from a wider perspective than evaluation through, for example, considering whether these are the *right* activities in the first place (are the aims and objectives appropriate, acceptable to all those concerned; would other activities provide better value for money or bigger health gains?). Audit may focus not only on the programmes, services and projects which an organization or alliance implements, but also considers whether there are important areas for which the organization/alliance has responsibility and in which it has failed to take action. Audit *compares* activities with similar activities undertaken elsewhere, in order to identify how performance could be improved (for example, through

continued on next page

continued

comparing quality standards with nationally accepted ones). Audit also focuses on whether *managerial systems* are in place to assure and continuously improve the quality of activities, and to ensure probity (ensuring that monies are used properly) and legality (ensuring that legal powers are not exceeded). It could *focus on one particular viewpoint* (for instance, on whether the activities of an organization or alliance meet the requirements of local people, or service users, through an audit of their preferences and views). It could also look at whether the balance of activities, carried out by an organization, is congruent with the overall purpose, goals and values of the organization (for example, through identifying whether certain high-priority health promotion issues are relatively neglected or whether access to health promotion for certain priority client groups is relatively restricted). Audit *results* (outputs) could be used not only to develop providers' quality improvement management systems, and to inform service specifications, but also to help purchasers to decide whether to renew or award contracts to health promotion providers. It is important to note that audit is *not* about judging the performance of individual people. *Peer appraisal* can contribute to audit, through focusing on the management and performance of people carrying out health promotion work. The purpose of peer appraisal is not to judge or criticize each other, but to improve the people management systems so that these provide the support and encouragement staff need in order continually to improve performance. All forms of audit are thus *development* processes, with the end goal (in health promotion work) of *health development*: developing healthy organizations, healthy alliances, healthy staff and healthy clients/service users.

Evaluation

Evaluation involves making a judgement about the value of something—in our case, about the value of a particular health promotion activity (1). Evaluation focuses exclusively on one particular activity, or project, which is its concern. Evaluation is the process of making a detailed assessment about what has been achieved and how it has been achieved. It means looking critically at the activity or project, working out what was good about it, what was bad about it, and how it could be improved.

The judgement can be about the *outcome* (what has been achieved)—whether the activity achieved the objectives which were set. So, for example, it could be about whether people understood the recommended limits for alcohol consumption as a result of your "sensible drinking" education, whether people in a particular community became more articulate about their health needs as a result of your community development work, or whether you achieved media coverage for your campaign.

Judgement can also be about the *process* (how it has been achieved): whether the most appropriate methods were used, whether they were used in the most effective way, and whether they gave value for money. So, for

continued on next page

continued

example, it could be about considering whether the video-based discussion used in a teaching programme was the best teaching method to use; whether the community development approach you chose for a programme was the most appropriate one in the circumstances; or whether more public awareness would have been achieved with less money if the promotion of your programme had opted for a media "stunt" with possible free news coverage rather than an expensive advertising and leaflet campaign. (Evaluation is discussed in more depth in Chapter 6.)

The concerns of audit and research and evaluation therefore overlap and an audit will make use of relevant research and evaluation documents and other management data.

WHY AUDIT OF HEALTH PROMOTION IS NECESSARY

Despite the increased emphasis on audit of public sector activities in recent years, there is little evidence of comprehensive systems to audit the very wide range of activities and policies subsumed under the umbrella of health promotion. The reason for this may be the complexity of attempting to audit the activities of a whole range of agencies, such as health authorities and trusts, specialist health promotion services, local authorities, primary care providers, GPs, schools, businesses and voluntary agencies, who are working together at local level on various aspects of health promotion. While the local specialist health promotion service may perform a coordinating role, no one agent or agency alone can be held accountable for the outcomes of the activities of a complex network of partnerships. Yet with the setting of targets for *The Health of the Nation* (and for corresponding strategies in other parts of the UK) it is essential that health promotion activities are subjected to as close a scrutiny as other work aiming to improve health. We must be able to demonstrate that we are avoiding duplication and waste of resources, whichever agency is involved, that we are moving forward in a concerted way towards long-term goals and targets, and that we are accountable for the work we do. We must therefore grasp this nettle, and below I make some suggestions about how this could be done. However, it is important to note that those organizations and alliances which have already developed good-quality management systems, such as those described in Chapter 4, will have collected all or most of the information required for an audit, and the audit task will be greatly simplified. On the other hand, organizations and alliances which have not yet developed quality improvement systems could begin with an audit to act as a catalyst for starting the process (for example, through helping to identify what quality systems are needed).

The benefits of audit of health promotion

- Audit helps with establishing good-quality improvement systems.
- Health promotion providers will further develop and improve their own internal quality improvement management systems.
- Purchasers will get assurance of the quality of the health promotion services provided through verification of their quality systems and management processes and through, for example, evidence that services provide "value for money", or evidence that activities are congruent with strategic goals and objectives.
- Staff morale will be improved through highlighting areas of good practice, and through using their own ideas to improve health promotion work.
- Better communication across all staff groups and professions, and with managers, resulting in a shared sense of purpose and a better understanding of health promotion.
- Improved collaboration and cooperation both within teams and across teams.
- An enhanced profile for health promotion locally.
- The spread of audit will contribute towards agreements on nationally approved standards for health-promoting organizations and for health promotion services and programmes, which will further stimulate quality in health promotion.

HOW TO CONDUCT A HEALTH PROMOTION AUDIT

I suggest that one approach to audit of health promotion work could be to conduct it on a *programme* basis. By a programme I mean a substantial and continuing body of local activities designed to fulfil particular strategic goals and targets related to a local priority, such as one of *The Health of the Nation* key areas (for example, an HIV/AIDS and sexual health programme, or a smoking control programme, or a heart health programme). A programme could be audited through scrutinizing the contributions of each separate agency, or through scrutinizing the joint working of a number of agencies (who are together providing a programme in a *health alliance*). *Projects, services* and *promotions* are the activities which together make up a programme.

- *Projects* are time-limited and the nature of projects varies over time, providing stepping stones towards the strategic goals.
- *Services* are continuing provisions, such as screening clinics, or leisure and recreation services, or health education courses, which make an integral contribution to programmes.
- *Promotions* are publicity and marketing events which raise awareness of the programme.
- *Policies, protocols* and *procedures* may provide guidance and direction on how the services and projects will operate.
- *Training* and *staff development* may be an integral component of the programme, ensuring the quality of activities.

The starting point for audit could therefore be to identify all the current provisions (projects, services, promotions and related policies, procedures and training) which contribute to a particular programme in a particular locality (city, county, etc.). An example is set out in the following box.

A smoking control programme

A local smoking control programme might include:

- *Non-smoking environments*: pubs, restaurants, hospitals, public transport, workplaces, schools, etc.
- *Smoking cessation services*: counselling, advisory services, etc.
- *Policies*: of health authorities, NHS trusts, local authorities, local businesses, schools, colleges, etc.
- *Local projects*: for vulnerable groups of people, or disadvantaged communities, etc.
- *Promotions and publicity*: projects in partnership with local mass media; special events and exhibitions, etc.
- *Staff training*: training in counselling skills, and in methods of helping people to change lifestyles and stop smoking.

This could then be analysed in terms of:

- *Who* provides each item? (Which agents and agencies?)
- *How many*?
- *Where*?
- *To what quality*? (What is the evidence about effectiveness, economy, efficiency, acceptability to users and ethical considerations?)

A picture would then emerge, providing evidence of gaps or duplication of services/projects, etc., needs for improved access to services and areas for improvement. The hardest question to answer will inevitably be the one about quality. In order to do this it will be necessary to gather information from three sources:

- *Comparative* information, such as standards set in other geographical areas or by other organizations, which can be compared with the standards set by the programme under investigation.
- *Normative* information from a range of professions and disciplines with a role in health promotion (normative information is information described by an expert or professional according to his or her standards).
- Information about *perceived needs, wants and preferences* from local people themselves.

Attempting something like this is potentially a huge job, and the problem can be knowing where to start. It will be essential to divide this up into bite-sized chunks. It will only be possible, in practice, to fill in one piece of the "jigsaw" at a time. Any agency or alliance contributing to health promotion and contemplating undertaking audit activities will need, first, to identify criteria about what to audit and when (this is discussed further in a later section of this chapter).

An alternative approach to tackling audit on a programme basis, could be to tackle it on an *organizational* basis, and look at a particular organization's ability to provide high-quality health promotion services and interventions. This would involve scrutinizing the health promotion work of a particular department, team, service or directorate, or of a whole organization. This could be done through a separate health promotion audit, or, when the work of an organization is audited, the health promotion components could be audited alongside, for example, clinical activities. The sorts of issues which such an audit might focus on include:

- Quality of mission statement, policy and planning framework (strategic management).
- Quality of organizational structure and health promotion management processes (operational management).
- Quality of resources for health promotion work (especially human resources).
- Health promotion quality improvement systems (quality management).
- Quality of information and communication systems and relationships (communications and relationships contributing to coordination, integration and the spread of innovations).

Audit methods

The sort of *methods* which could be used include:

- Gathering information from existing documents (such as project information and evaluation reports, planning documents, records of quality improvement systems, activity data, service specifications and standards).
- In-depth interviews, conducted by a skilled interviewer, with staff at all levels and grades including directors, managers, team leaders, team members and all professions and occupations contributing to the work of the organization, using predetermined structured questions.
- Focus groups (discussions with groups of staff, or with service users, focusing on predetermined questions).
- Peer-conducted interviews (staff performing the same or similar roles interviewing each other in pairs, using predetermined structured questions).
- Gathering information from regular observations and monitoring of project/service delivery (such as observations on smoking in non-smoking areas).
- Questionnaires.

Who should conduct health promotion audits?

I have now, hopefully, made some suggestions which will help audit of health promotion work to be carried out. An equally important point is, *who* should carry out this audit? Because health promotion work is multidisciplinary, I believe that audit should ideally be carried out by a multidisciplinary team, with representation from all the professions and disciplines involved in the health promotion work concerned. This audit team will often be a group of staff who work for the organization concerned (an *internal audit team*). It would be wise, when first attempting an audit, for the team either to include an *outsider* (an independent facilitator or consultant, perhaps from another geographical area, with health promotion research/evaluation/audit expertise, who has no connection with the programme or organization, in order to avoid bias, and to provide help which ensures an objective scrutiny), or to have access to supervision and support from an external facilitator.

In order to be effective, such internal audit teams will require training, ultimately possibly leading to accreditation. The sort of training needs which will emerge include training in devising unbiased, structured questions, training in interviewing skills, training in groupwork, for conducting focus groups, training in the skills of peer appraisal, and training in how to compile audit reports. The assurance of confidentiality is a key issue at all stages of the audit process (without this core condition any audit will be worthless), and how to build in structures and processes which support confidentiality will be a key aspect of the training. Who could provide this? The Audit Commission is one obvious body to look to for help and support. Another possibility could be that a "National Health Promotion Quality/Audit Council" is set up to train and supervise health promotion auditors. All this, of course, would require paying for! Health authorities (or health commissions formed by mergers of health authorities and family health services authorities) could be given a (possibly statutory) responsibility to arrange for, and fund, audits of local health promotion work, and could be obliged to employ trained and accredited auditors. (For a discussion on quality improvement training, of which audit training forms a part, see Chapter 4.)

At present, external facilitation is a necessary element of any internal audit scheme, to help with supervision, training and data collection. The exact role the facilitator will play will depend on local factors, such as what skills a particular facilitator has to offer, what are the needs of the local audit team, and what finance is available.

One existing scheme for auditing health promotion work has been developed by the Society of Health Education and Health Promotion Specialists (2). It is based on a form of "external audit". A set of guidelines has been produced for use by experienced health promotion specialists (auditors who act as external facilitators) who have received training in the use of the guidelines. The guidelines are designed to reflect good practice back to auditees and to expose any weaknesses, deficiencies or inconsistencies in the quality management systems. The guidelines provide a framework to classify the mechanisms by which a department or team reviews their own work performance (the role of the "auditor" is thus to facilitate and support self-audit). This scheme is open to specialist health promotion services/departments. Wider schemes open to any organization, department, service, team or alliance with a health promotion role have yet to be established.

District Audit (the main external auditors of the NHS) have recently undertaken a "value for money" audit at Rotherham Health Promotion Unit (3). This focused on a number of key questions which are set out in an adapted format as follows:

Questions to ask when conducting a health promotion organizational audit

Strategic planning issues: scrutinizing key documentation and holding key discussions to establish whether the unit:

- Has a clear understanding of its purpose and objectives.
- Has taken on board external strategic influences (such as *The Health of the Nation*).

continued on next page

continued

- Has policies and programmes based on a good knowledge of local health needs.
- Has intentions consistent with the health promotion strategies set by purchasers/providers and other local agencies, such as the local authority.
- Is actively involved in the development of purchaser and provider health promotion strategy, through making a contribution to strategic plans?

Operational planning issues: scrutinizing key documentation and holding key discussions to establish whether the unit:

- Has annual plans which are consistent with the overall health promotion strategy.
- Involves all its staff in the development of annual plans.
- Consults with other agencies and local people about annual plans.
- Clearly defines the responsibilities of individual staff, in terms of the contribution they will make to implementing annual plans.
- Ensures that tasks are prioritized and timetabled.
- Measures its performance in all key areas.
- Assesses and reports the results of interventions.
- Promotes ("sells") its performance to purchasers and other key local agencies.

Staffing issues: scrutinizing key documentation and holding key discussions to establish whether the unit:

- Determines the staff numbers, grades and skill mix required to carry out plans.
- Organizes the workload efficiently, for example so that work is spread equitably.
- Provides effective supervision and control of staff performance (through support, help and encouragement by supervisors and managers).
- Recognizes and meets the training and development needs of staff.
- Conducts upward appraisal (has mechanisms for ensuring that staff perceptions on the performance of supervisors and managers are listened to and acted on when appropriate).
- Has good systems for managing its human resources (recruitment, retention, equal opportunities, etc.).

Relationship issues: scrutinizing key documentation and holding key discussions to establish whether the unit:

- Has adequate contact with other agencies in order to ensure coordination of effort with other agencies.
- Has established relationships which ensure a high level of awareness of health promotion within its own authority.
- Has good systems for reporting to its own authority, ensuring approval of plans and reporting of activities.

continued on next page

continued

Communication issues: scrutinizing key documentation and holding key discussions to establish whether the unit:

- Disseminates good practice to others through contributing to local and national networks and publications.
- Publicizes its activities in a way which is easily understood by local people in order to ensure accountability to local people
- Builds contacts with the local business community in order to work in partnership with them.

Any organization involved in health promotion can use or adapt these questions, to contribute to an internal organizational audit.

In addition, Trent Regional Health Authority have been attempting to develop models of practice for audit of health promotion services, through audit activities at three sites within the region (Nottingham Health Development Directorate, Doncaster Health Promotion Department and Sheffield Health Promotion Directorate) (4). Doncaster Health Promotion Department have designed a developmental approach to audit, which is concerned with the gradual introduction of quality ideas and methods and focuses as much on managerial quality and quality of participation by local people as on professional quality (these are the three key dimensions of quality which are focused on in the quality improvement management system which I discuss in Chapter 4). They have used an approach to mapping and analysing a health promotion client's path through the health promotion service, from selection and entry, to closure and follow-up, in order to identify ways of improving quality. This is based on an approach to audit recently advocated by John Øvretveit, for application to any health service (5).

The Cancer Relief Macmillan Fund recently launched an organizational audit specifically designed for those organizations working in palliative care (6). It combines a framework of nationally approved standards covering issues which are consistent across all palliative care settings, with the identification of good practice and areas for improvement. The system has been tested in a number of key settings, and was developed with the advice and cooperation of the King's Fund Organizational Audit Unit. The average cost for the audit over a year is £6500, which includes intensive training and the services of a survey manager throughout the period as well as the survey itself. This system could provide some pointers for the development of "quality" health promotion audit systems.

Getting started

In the meantime, it is up to those organizations involved in health promotion work to invest in and to spread audit. For example, health promotion partnerships (health alliances) could agree to undertake audit of key aspects of their programmes. Training could be commissioned for the auditors. To do this, of course, takes time and costs money, and it is important to weigh the costs of audit against the validity and usefulness of the information it provides. As I previously pointed out, the better the existing quality management systems of organizations or agencies forming an alliance, the easier it will be to audit the health promotion work, and thus valuable time and resources will not be wasted. It is also essential to have some clear criteria about *what to audit, and when, and in how much detail.* The sort of criteria you might want to use are set out in the following box.

Criteria about what to audit, and when

- *Management concern*: for example, health gain not achieved; many agencies or teams working together; poor communication or low morale.
- *Expensive*: for example, lack of information about whether activities provide value for money.
- *Demonstrable*: for example, activity can be measured; standards, outputs and outcomes can be demonstrated to stakeholders.
- *Practical*: for example, expert audit facilitators available, commitment of auditees; finance available.
- *Principles and values*: for example, to clarify whether the values and principles expressed in your mission statement (or the philosophies of an alliance) are realized; ethical considerations.
- *Expressed need*: acknowledgement of the need to establish or further develop quality improvement systems.

GUIDELINES FOR CONDUCTING AN AUDIT

1. Start with a small, low-cost scheme, in order to establish whether investment in audit is worthwhile and how best to introduce it.
2. Select a leader for the audit project with great care (the ability to build relationships with staff and managers at all levels, based on mutual respect and trust is crucial).
3. Provide the leader with support (for example, from an external facilitator).
4. Use volunteers for membership of the audit team, and ensure that the team is drawn from across all professions, occupations, grades and

levels of staff, and from across all sites (if work is based at a number of different sites).

5. Identify the training needs of the audit team, and establish how the training could best be provided. (See the sections on "Quality management of people" and "The role of the manager in professional development" in Chapter 4, for a discussion on some of the skills needed and on the principles of quality improvement training.)
6. Ensure that the audit team have the time to carry out the proposed activities (time for training, gathering key documents, conducting interviews, writing reports, developing new quality improvement systems, etc.).
7. Prepare the ground before audit activities start, in order to allay anxieties and fears. Establish ground rules (voluntary participation in audit activities, through "informed consent", the right to "pass" on any question, how confidentiality will be maintained).
8. Establish how the audit will be evaluated and reported on right from the start, so that the necessary information can be gathered as you go along. It may be necessary to produce several reports for different audiences and purposes. For example:
   - An evaluation of the audit processes and outcomes will be necessary, so that you know how best to audit next time, and so that you identify all the outcomes of the audit, both intended and unintended.
   - You may wish to publish this evaluation, in order to spread good audit practice.
   - In addition, you will need to report on the findings and recommendations of the audit, and to describe the steps which are required to establish or improve quality systems.
   - The findings and recommendations may need to be reported at different levels. For example, to the organization itself, for internal action. Thus, some of the audit tools may be suitable for modification in order to incorporate them into the quality system on a regular ongoing basis (for example, focus groups could become ongoing quality circles; peer-conducted interviews could become an ongoing way of offering each other mutual support). Some changes may have costs, in terms of money. The organization itself, or the purchaser, may need to consider and decide how to act on these recommendations.
   - You may also wish to report the findings to other stakeholders, such as the local health commission, or the local authority, or other agencies. If so, you will need to consider what information will be required by these agencies, and how it could best be presented.
   - You may wish to report separately on the training components of your activities. Educational and development tools may be one outcome of an audit.

Accountability

Finally, one aim of audit is to improve *accountability*. This raises the question of "To whom should audit reports be made available?" There is no doubt in my mind that these should be made widely available to the general public, as well as to all the stakeholders (the agents and agencies concerned). Successful health promotion programmes aim to shape and influence behaviour, practices and policies at all levels in a locality—individual, group, organizational and community-wide. These far-reaching objectives mean that local agents and agencies must be held accountable not only for achieving the objectives of their programmes in the most cost-effective ways, but also that these are the *right* programmes, based on policies which will realistically contribute to health gain for local communities. The more local people can be actively involved in the scrutiny of health promotion, and in the shaping of policies and plans, the better (more successful) will be the direction of policy. It is therefore important that audit reports are produced in a language that local people can understand, and that they are widely publicized and made widely available (for example, through the media, and in public libraries). Audit reports can thus contribute to raising the profile of health promotion work at local level. Another approach could be to train "lay" volunteers to audit the views of local people about their health promotion needs and how these might best be met. This has the added value of enhancing community participation. However, this needs to be approached very sensitively, because local communities may not want their problems to be highlighted to all and sundry.

For more information on audit, see the note at the end of this chapter (7). The following case study, based on carrying out an audit of health promotion work in practice, was contributed by Dr Elizabeth Perkins and describes auditing health promotion activity in Nottingham. Her role was to facilitate audit of the work of the specialist Nottingham Health Development Directorate and was commissioned by Trent Regional Health Authority (8).

Auditing health promotion activity in Nottingham

Starting points

"Trent Health provided funding, through its Regional Health Promotion Officer, for the development of experimental internal audit projects. The Nottingham project, in a provider unit, has worked from a number of assumptions:

- Specific issues are best for audit (confirmed in the experience of medical audit).

continued on next page

continued

- Those issues should be a matter of concern to as many participants as possible.
- Outside help to set up an audit system is an efficient way to start.
- Approaches which rely on outside help for their maintenance may rapidly become unworkable because resources are not available to service this.

Nottingham Health Development Directorate wanted to improve its activity data collection system, which lacked a precise focus on *Health of the Nation* priorities. Discussion with purchasers was not helped by the limitations of the data, and staff disliked filling in forms which in subtle ways did not reflect the nature of their work. Altering the system was essential before activity data could be used to conduct a serious professional examination of the pattern of work in three very different teams: a group of specialist health promotion officers, a health centre team providing both a drop-in information service and an outreach approach centring on women's health, and the HIV team. Accordingly, a consultant was approached to work with staff to redesign the data collection system within the framework of audit.

Developing activity data

Work on this started in December 1993. The existing system provided a very useful focus for discussions, both on an individual basis and with groups, about the ways in which current work should be classified, and the process of piloting a new system was used both to improve its internal logic and to build in staff groups a sense of common understanding of the way in which categories should be used. As had been hoped, a sense of ownership of the system and the results has emerged alongside the improvements. The new system was in place, as planned, for the start of the new financial year, and has been computerized through the shareware package Epi-info.

Learning to use the data

The first two audit meetings were held in July and October, with each team separately. The results received a good reception, including requests for each individual's three-monthly totals for use in self-monitoring. Health promotion specialists were encouraged to compare their expectations of the distribution of the department's work with the figures for the last three months; after some initial hesitations, this produced fruitful discussion, including a recognition of their limited

continued on next page

continued

knowledge of the work of the other teams, and sometimes even of colleagues in the same team. The data encouraged a wider view of professional practice, as a product of the whole service, rather than as an individual affair. At this stage, staff were more interested in the whole picture than in individual programmes, though it was recognized that it will be helpful in future to use the facility to pull out data on one or other of *The Health of the Nation* targets or settings, in relation to client groups or types of activities. It has been agreed that meetings should continue on a three-monthly basis but be held jointly, to enable discussion of the work of the service as a whole.

The development of audit

The audit cycle, once an issue has been identified, normally starts with the specification of standards or criteria, followed by the collection of data, the assessment of performance, and the identification of a need for change. In this it closely resembles the quality cycle. It is in the nature of cycles, however, that one can start anywhere. There are no norms concerning the proper distribution of professional time, as with many issues in health promotion. Using the new data, Nottingham health promotion specialists are proposing to develop their own norms, with appropriate consultation with their purchasers. As ideas emerge and are refined, they can be checked against the data and practice can be adapted if appropriate. At the same time Nottingham health promotion specialists are now taking a much more active approach to internal quality monitoring, moving beyond the basic issues tackled with all services in the Trust to pick up matters of more concern in health promotion. There seems to be considerable scope for further development through the linked processes of audit and quality, now that they are viewed as matters for staff initiative on areas of their choice, rather than as potentially tedious organizational demands which distract people from useful work.

There are a number of ways in which it has been suggested that audit processes and findings can be shared between Specialist Health Promotion Services. This project has been designed to produce a transferable, and adaptable, tool. The activity data collection system, a computer disk, and guidance notes for the introduction of the system and on its use in audit based on experience so far, are expected to be available by the end of 1994. If this is of interest to other services, the sharing of results will become a possibility in future, subject to the issues about commercial confidentiality which increasingly bedevil exchange of experience on good practice in the health service."

Elizabeth R. Perkins
November 1994

To sum up, audit can not only be a way of improving the performance of particular aspects of health promotion work, it can also be a starting point for reflecting on quality, and for gaining experience in how to develop effective quality improvement management systems.

Questions you could ask yourself

1. Using the criteria about what to audit, and when, plus any additional criteria you think are important, identify which specific aspects of the health promotion work of your organization (or of an alliance you contribute to) would benefit from an audit. Then think about *who* could conduct the audit, *how* it could be financed, *what* it would focus on, *what methods* could be employed to collect the audit information, *when* it would be best to carry it out, *what training* would be required, and *to whom* the outputs would be made available. Finally, consider what steps you could take to enable this to happen.
2. Think about how you could use the information about audit in this chapter, to improve the way you routinely review and improve the health promotion work of your business, organization, department, service or unit.

NOTES, REFERENCES AND FURTHER READING

(1) This section is based on a discussion of evaluation in:

Ewles, L. and Simnett, I. (3rd edn, 1995) *Promoting Health: A Practical Guide*. London: Scutari Press. Ch. 6.

(2) The Society of Health Education and Health Promotion Specialists' audit scheme runs informally, with requests for audit visits being referred to one of a list of trained auditors. The focus of each audit is agreed between participants, along with practical arrangements and any costs to be levied. The auditor and auditee are asked to provide a brief report for quality monitoring and training purposes. For more information on the scheme, contact:

Brian Neeson, North and Mid Hampshire Health Commission, Harness House, Aldermaston Road, Basingstoke RG24 9NB. Telephone: 01256 312252.

(3) For further information contact Rotherham Health Promotion Service, 1–2 Chatham Villas, Chatham Street, Rotherham, South Yorks S65 1DP. Telephone: 01709 820020. For information on local "value for money" audit contact your local District Audit Service.

(4) For further information contact Rae Magowan, Trent Regional Health of the Nation Coordinator, Fulwood House, Old Fulwood Road, Sheffield S10 3TH. Telephone: 01742 630300.

The Sheffield Health Promotion Directorate have produced a report on the process, methods and learning from the Sheffield Health Promotion Audit and an "Audit Tool-Kit", which can be obtained from:

Sheffield Centre for HIV and Sexual Health, 22 Collegiate Crescent, Sheffield S10 2BA. Telephone: 01114 267 8806.

Kevin Blanks has produced a report on the Doncaster Health Promotion audit process. This can be obtained from Doncaster Health Promotion Department, Alverley Lodge, St Catherine's Hospital, Tickhill Road, Doncaster DN4 8QN. Telephone: 01302 854661.

Elizabeth Perkins has produced a report on the Health Promotion Activity Audit in Nottingham. This can be obtained from Elizabeth R. Perkins, 11 Exton Road, Sherwood, Nottingham NG5 1HA. Telephone: 0115 9609 098.

(5) Øvretveit, J. (1994) Roads to Recovery. *Health Service Journal* **104** (5407): 32–33.

(6) For further information contact Marney Prouse, Organizational Audit Programme Manager, Cancer Relief Macmillan Fund, 11 Elvaston Place, London SW7 5QG. Telephone: 0171 589 9160.

(7) See, for example:

Audit Commission (1993) *Putting Quality on the Map: Measuring and Appraising Quality in the Public Service.* Occasional Paper No. 18. London: Audit Commission.

The volume on *Quality Issues in Health-Promotion Work,* which is part of the *Managing Health Improvement Project* (MAHIP) open learning material, contains a unit on "Audit of Health-Promotion Work", which was written by Ina Simnett. For information about the availability of these materials, see note (8) at the end of chapter 1.

For a recent article on auditing health promotion, see:

Catford, J. (1993) Auditing health promotion: what are the vital signs of quality. *Health Promotion International* **8** (2): 67–68.

For an introduction to medical audit in primary health care, see:

Lawrence, M. and Schofield, T. (eds) (1993) *Medical Audit in Primary Health Care.* Oxford: Oxford University Press. GP Series No. 25.

(8) This case study was written by Elizabeth Perkins and is reproduced by kind permission of Nottingham Community Health NHS Trust.

CHAPTER 6 Setting goals and objectives and measuring achievements of health promotion

Summary

The chapter begins by looking at national and local health strategies and at the emergence of joint health strategies (strategies which are shared by a number of different agencies at local level). A case study provides an example of how agencies are working to a common agenda in one London borough. The next section identifies what is meant by goals, objectives and targets, and discusses how different types of objectives and targets are needed in health promotion work. This leads on to a discussion about evaluation (how to measure progress towards targets), including a discussion on the importance of knowing why you are evaluating and to whom the evaluation will be made available. Ways of measuring both processes and outcomes are suggested. The final section briefly touches on the final stage of the health gain spiral—review—and discusses the contribution of health economics to making judgements about how best to use scarce resources. The chapter ends with an activity you could undertake in order to form judgements about national and local health strategies, and some questions you could ask yourself to help you to improve your evaluations.

This chapter focuses on three key aspects of managing for health gain: first, the need for a strategic approach at both national and local levels, which sets the scene for working together and detailed planning; second, the need for setting realistic and achievable goals, objectives and targets; third, the importance of evaluation and review, so that achievements are measured, ways to improve performance are identified and the best use is made of resources. Some of the terms in common usage related to planning and evaluation are defined in a note at the end of the chapter (1).

HEALTH STRATEGIES

For the first time, we now have national strategies for health (as opposed to strategies for health *services*), with a clear emphasis on planning for improving, maintaining and restoring *health,* as opposed to just planning for the provision of health and social care and treatment services. Health promotion has a key part to play in these strategies, although effective treatment and care continue, of course, to play a part. Health gain has become one focus of the prime mission of the NHS, along with the provision of high-quality treatment and care. The role of health authorities has been reoriented towards improving the health of the population for whom they are responsible.

The four UK national health strategy documents differ in some respects (2). England's *The Health of the Nation* has been criticized for largely failing to acknowledge the socio-economic determinants of health. It mentions inequalities as "variations" in health status (3) and looks to the lifestyle change model of health promotion as the way forward. The Welsh strategy takes a broader view, and includes "emotional health and relationships", "physical disability" and "healthy environments" in its priorities for action. Its strategy documents identify the "health skills" required to safeguard health and lead socially fulfilling lives: knowledge, attitudes, self-confidence, coping and relationships, parenting, safety and first aid, self-help and mutual support. Scotland's strategy emphasizes the importance of environmental factors, and the Northern Ireland strategy includes discussion of the impact of "material deprivation" on health. All four, however, emphasize lifestyle factors, such as smoking, drinking and sexual behaviour, as crucial.

More recently, the Republic of Ireland has announced a health strategy which is more all-embracing than any of the UK ones (4). The strategy identifies equity, quality and accountability as its guiding principles. It has a clear sense of purpose—health and social gain with equity at the fore—and establishes clear health gain targets. Instead of building a health service market, as has happened in the UK, it suggests that the organizational arrangements best suited to achieving improved health and enhanced quality and equity are a closer integration of hospital and community services. By avoiding national prescriptions for organizational change it gives local health and social services, and local people, the opportunity, and the responsibility, to shape their own futures.

Local health strategies

A local health strategy is based on an assessment of local needs and an understanding of the local factors which contribute towards better health or cause ill-health. It is also based on an assessment of those things which a health commissioner can influence in order to improve health, and an understanding of the part which could be played by a wide range of local agents and agencies in achieving health gain. As a result of these assessments, health commissioners make decisions about the types, range and balance of interventions which have the prospects of achieving the greatest health gain.

The health strategy of an organization consists of a mission and goals, objectives and targets, unique to that organization. (I explain what is meant by these terms in the next section of this chapter, but we are talking about specifying, in increasing levels of detail, what health gains an organization aspires to achieve.) Most statutory agencies at a local level (district health authorities or health boards, health commissions formed by mergers of Health Authorities and Family Health Services Authorities, or local authorities) have produced their own local health strategies which fit in with national strategies. (For a discussion on the steps needed to formulate local health strategies, see the section on "Commissioning: formulating health strategy and programmes" in Chapter 3.) In England, for example, district health authorities have set their own local targets for the key areas specified in *The Health of the Nation*. They are also required to monitor their achievement of the targets.

Joint health strategies and joint commissioning

Many health commissions, local authorities and other local agencies are now working towards *joint* health strategies. A joint health strategy is a statement for the *collaboration* between different organizations, with shared objectives for achieving health gain. Each of the collaborating organizations will also have its own unique objectives. The joint strategy may involve partners agreeing to take delegated responsibility for certain objectives, or for purchasing or providing appropriate programmes or services. It could also involve sharing resources, jointly commissioning services or programmes, which could be jointly managed by the relevant provider agencies and involve joint working by front-line staff. In this context we can make a distinction between coordination, cooperation and collaboration (5).

- *Coordination* is a broad term involving all those situations where an organization aims to ensure that its own activities take into account those of others.
- *Cooperation* happens when organizations interact so that each may achieve its own objectives better.
- *Collaboration* describes the situation where participants work together to pursue a joint strategy, with shared objectives, while also pursuing their own individual objectives.

Health alliances are examples of cooperation and/or collaboration.

Fundamentally, any joint health strategy will have three key aspects:

1. *Working together*: All purchasers, whether health authorities, family health services authorities (FHSAs), GP fundholders or local authorities, will need to work together in a concerted way, in order to develop and design a joint strategy.
2. *In identified key areas*: purchasers must tackle health problems and improve health through working in a number of key (priority) programme areas. These include:
   - *Health promotion*: preventing ill-health, health education to promote better health, and health protection through making "healthy choices the easier choices". Examples include:
     - For individuals, measures such as preventing disease through immunization; screening to find and treat early stages of disease; health education to promote healthy lifestyles.
     - For communities, measures such as ensuring safe food, safe and healthy environments, no-smoking policies in workplaces, and "drink–driving" legislation.
   - *Diagnosing and treating ill-health and disease*: this includes personal medical treatment both in primary and secondary care. It is aimed at diagnosis of disease, treatment where appropriate, and rehabilitation of those with ongoing problems so as to minimize potential handicaps.
   - *Caring for people who are ill, vulnerable or who have disabilities*: in circumstances where people cannot be cured or have disabilities or problems which require continuing care, care must be provided so that the individual and his or her carers can live as comfortable, independent and "normal" a life as possible, preferably in the location of their choice.
   - *Research and development and evaluation*: this is a prerequisite for ensuring that effective, appropriate, acceptable and cost-effective services and interventions are provided which are responsive to changing health and health promotion needs and to improvements in practices.
3. *According to a plan*: given the limit to available resources, purchasers will not be in a position to meet all of the identified needs. It is thus essential for district health authorities and FHSAs jointly to identify local priorities for action, in collaboration with other local agencies involved in health improvement. The establishment of plans by such health alliances can create a shared vision to:

   - Identify shared objectives and targets for action.
   - Develop joint strategies and plans.

- Determine lead responsibility for action.
- Jointly commission programmes, projects and services.
- Collaborate on implementing the plans.

Case study: joint commissioning and joint working in Bromley (6)

The statutory authorities in Bromley have a long history of joint working on health promotion and published a joint health promotion strategy in 1993. One project, "Healthy Crays", offers a good example of a joint initiative. The statutory and non-statutory agencies are working together to build a community-led healthy lifestyle programme in one of the more deprived parts of the borough.

Joint working has also received a major push with the transfer of community care responsibilities to the local authority. Joint working on health promotion and community care has been facilitated by a joint commissioning process developed in 1991 from the old joint consultative committee approach. In 1993 a review of joint commissioning resulted in new explicit agreements and terms of reference for joint commissioning, based on a realistic appraisal of levels of decision making and influence. In November 1993 Bromley council members and officers met for a conference with their counterparts from Bromley Health and NHS Trusts. Small mixed groups of health and local authority executives, officers, members and non-executive directors worked together to make connections between health and social issues. It was recognized that many differences exist between local authorities and health authorities and NHS Trusts, for example the planning and decision-making timetables are different. Nevertheless, the new joint commissioning strategy was recognized as offering opportunities for "scoring doubles" through economies of scale as well as through a broader view of how to influence the health and quality of life for all Bromley residents.

There have been further developments since the conference. The leader of the council and the chair of Bromley Health now meet regularly to discuss progress and this is mirrored in periodic joint meetings between the two authorities' management teams. Bromley Health's chief executive has been appointed a member of the Community Safety Panel, a multi-agency initiative promoted by Bromley council and police. These moves reinforce the appreciation of the extent of the common agenda being pursued by the statutory authorities.

SETTING GOALS AND OBJECTIVES FOR HEALTH PROMOTION (7)

People use a whole gamut of words to describe statements of "what we intend to achieve"—aims, objectives, targets, goals, mission, purpose, achievement, result, product, outcomes. Though there is no universal agreement about the precise meaning of these words, it can be helpful to think of them as forming a hierarchy. At the top of the hierarchy are words that tell you why your organization exists, such as its purpose or mission (8). In the middle of the hierarchy are words that describe what the organization plans to do in general terms, such as its goals or aims. At the bottom of the hierarchy are words that describe in specific detail what it intends to achieve, such as targets or objectives.

Objectives can be of different kinds. *Health* objectives are usually expressed as the outcome or end state to be achieved in terms of health status, such as reduced rates of illness or death. However, in health promotion work objectives are often expressed in terms of steps along the way towards an ultimate improvement in the health of individuals or populations ("staging posts"). For example, in health education work, *educational* objectives are framed in terms of the knowledge, attitudes or behaviour to be exhibited by the learner as the outcome of the education. Objectives can also be in terms of *other kinds of changes,* such as a change in health policy (for example, introducing a no-smoking policy in a workplace), or changes in social or environmental conditions (for example, the provision of safe areas for children to play in and take physical exercise), or in health promotion practices (for example, providing health information in minority ethnic languages or establishing a coronary rehabilitation programme).

The term "targets" is increasingly used in national and local documents. Targets usually specify how the achievement of an objective will be *measured,* in terms of quantity, quality, and time (the date by which the objective will be achieved). Thus, a *health target* can be defined as a measurable improvement in health status, by a given time, which achieves a health objective. This is the approach used in *The Health of the Nation* national strategy for health in England: the objectives are framed as *health* objectives, and the targets are framed as *health targets* (changes in rates of death or illness by a specific date) or *behaviour targets* (such as changes in smoking or drinking by a specific date).

Targets can be set at all levels, from the national level, the local (for example, city or county) level, the locality (neighbourhood) level, down to the level of the individual service user or client.

Criteria have been suggested for the design and specification of high-quality targets (9).

SMART criteria for specifying targets

S Specific (to a disease, a risk factor, a social group, an age, a sex, an ethnic group, or a geographical location).

M Measurable (using important indicators, not just "measuring the measurable").
A Agreed (by all concerned, for example all the members of an alliance, the public).
R Realistic (achievable within resource and other constraints).
T Timebound (achievable within a time-scale).

Setting health gain targets at local level is a complex task, partly because of the small numbers sometimes making it difficult to measure progress towards health outcomes. Commissioning agencies must make judgements about *progress targets* ("staging posts") which will lead to the overall achievement of long-term local health objectives.

EVALUATION AND REVIEW OF HEALTH PROMOTION (10)

How will you know whether the health promotion work you are responsible for managing is successful? And how will you measure success (11)? There are no easy answers to these crucial questions about evaluation. On a large scale, sophisticated research can be mounted. This should not deter you from ensuring that all health promotion activities are evaluated; modest methods of evaluating the everyday practice of health promotion can, and should, be used routinely. The sorts of key questions which your evaluation is designed to answer include:

- Did you achieve your objectives and, if not, why not?
- Were the resources used to best effect?
- Were their any unexpected spin-offs?
- What should you do next?

Defining terms

What is meant by "evaluation"? Simply, making a judgement about the value of something—in this case, about the value of health promotion work, whether it is implementing a health promotion programme, for example, or a community development project, or the development of a local policy, or environmental changes, or organizational changes which will have an impact on health. Evaluation is the process of assessing what has been achieved (whether the specified goals, objectives and targets have been met) and how it has been achieved. It means looking critically at the intervention, working out what was good about it, what was bad about it, and how it could be improved.

The judgement can be about the *outcome* (what has been achieved)—whether you achieved the objectives which you set. Judgement can also be about the *process* (how it has been achieved)—whether the most appropriate methods were used, whether they were used in the most effective way, and whether they gave value for money.

Why evaluate?

The evaluation methods chosen and the data collected should always be a function of the *purpose* to which data are to be put. It is therefore essential to be clear about *why* health promotion work is being evaluated, because this will affect what is done and the amount of effort put into it.

Some reasons could be:

1. To improve local health promotion practice: next time something similar is done, it will be possible to build on past successes and learn the lessons from any mistakes (for example, through showing that a particular approach is more efficient or through improving materials or methods).
2. To spread good practice through helping other people to improve their practice: if you tell other people about your local experiences, it can help them to improve their practice as well.
3. To maximize the use of resources and to justify using the resources that went into the work for health promotion purposes (as opposed to using the resources for alternative activities).
4. To provide evidence to support the case for doing this work in the future (for example, evidence of effectiveness, through demonstrating that the work has the desired outcome). This sort of information is essential for future commissioning.
5. To give local professionals the satisfaction of knowing how useful or effective their work has been: in other words, to provide and improve motivation and job satisfaction.
6. To identify any aspects of the impact which were unplanned but could be important (for example, to identify unplanned benefits such as improved social well-being, self-esteem and relationships in a group of young single parents participating in a group to help them to stop smoking).
7. To assess whether the activities are ethically justifiable and to minimize any undesirable outcomes (for example, anxiety can be associated with some types of screening, and services need to take action to reduce it and/or help patients to cope with it).

Who for?

Who will be using the evaluation data? The answer to this affects what questions are asked, how much depth and detail are gone into and how to present the information.

If it is a report to purchasers/commissioners who you want to continue to fund the work, you need to think through what questions they will expect to be answered, and how much detail they will want.

For example, imagine you are the leader of a team of health visitors, midwives and physiotherapists, based at a local health centre, who are planning a pilot scheme for a new approach to parent education involving a drop-in advisory service for parents on certain evenings and an evening "phone-in" facility for those who cannot get to the health centre. Guidance will be provided for parents of children from all age groups from the antenatal period through childhood to adolescence, and links will be forged with other local professions and agencies providing services for young people, so that referrals can be made when appropriate. An evaluation report will be needed after six months by the Community Trust which has a contract with the local purchasing/ commissioning authority to provide the scheme. What will the Trust Board need to know? At the very least, they will probably need a clear indication of the use made of the scheme (who used it? how much? what for?), what the clients gained from it, and how much it cost. It may also be useful to compare the impact of the scheme with conventional approaches to parent education in similar localities, and with previous parent education in this locality. This will involve collecting data from other appropriate geographical areas, and historical data from your own locality. It may also be useful to look at the impact of the service on other local professions and agencies and their clients. This could involve interviewing other professions, including devising schedules for the interviews and for recording the findings. It would be helpful for you, as the team leader, to discuss with the health professionals what evaluation data will be required at the planning stage of the project, so that the appropriate data can be collected right from the start.

Evaluation of health promotion work falls into two broad categories:

- *Process* evaluation: this means looking at what goes on during the process of implementation, and making judgements about it. (Is it being done as cheaply and quickly as possible? Is the quality of the inputs and outputs as good as you want? Is it reaching those people for whom it is intended?)
- *Impact* and *outcome* evaluation: by impact I mean all the consequences of the health promotion work (including any unplanned consequences) and by outcome I mean whether you have achieved the planned objectives you set.

Evaluating the process

I turn first to evaluating the process. Process evaluation should take place in parallel with your implementation of a programme or project, so that you can immediately pick up any faults with the programme/project and rectify them straight away (in other words, it is a method of *quality control*). The sorts of questions to ask yourself include: Am I using appropriate methods and materials? Am I using resources efficiently? In other words, it is important to look at the management processes, as you go along, in order to assess how well you are performing.

How are you going to assess your performance? I suggest four key aspects: measuring the inputs, measuring progress on key performance indicators, self-evaluation by asking yourself questions, and getting feedback from other people.

- *Measuring the inputs* is essential if you are going to make judgements about whether the outcome was worthwhile. You need to record everything that went into your health promotion activity, in terms of time, staff, money, accommodation and materials. Then you can make an informed judgement about whether the outcome was worth the cost.
- *Performance indicators and progress targets*: by identifying important performance indicators and associated progress targets you can monitor and control your management performance. For example, a set of 12 indicators have been developed for *Health at Work in the NHS* along with progress targets (12). A description of one of these indicators (and the relevant progress targets) is set out in the following box.

Putting health at work into the performance management process (13)

Indicator

Development of management practices and monitoring systems across the organization to support positive health practices.

Progress targets

1. *Policies*: have you got policies to cover sickness and absenteeism, accident recording, labour turnover, appraisal, communication systems? Who has responsibility for these areas? Do personnel, health and safety, occupational health and specialist health promotion staff work together to develop effective health policies? Is the impact on health and well-being of all policies monitored and evaluated?

continued on next page

continued

2. *Sickness and absenteeism recording*: is there a system for collection of these data? Are these data analysed? Are data allocated to appropriate managers? Is a target set for reduction in sickness/absenteeism?
3. *Accident recording*: is there a system for recording these data? Are they analysed? Is there a system for recording "near misses"? Are these data fed to appropriate managers? Is a target for accident reduction set?
4. *Labour turnover*: is there a system for recording the number of exits each year? Is there an exit interview process? Is information fed back to managers? Is there a system for recording the number of ill-health early retirements each year? Are targets set to reduce turnover?
5. *Appraisal systems*: is there an appraisal or individual performance review system for each member of staff? Are management systems set up to examine regularly job, team, service and project specifications, organizational goals and objectives and workloads?
6. *Support and training*: are there support systems set up for staff in times of change? Is management and/or occupational training available for all grades of staff after needs have been identified?

To take another example, imagine you are participating in a health alliance to promote physical activity. The sort of performance indicators which you might decide to use include:

- Growth in active membership of local leisure and sports facilities.
- Opening of new sports and leisure clubs and facilities.
- Provision of new environments for physical activity such as play spaces.
- Numbers of people regularly attending sports and leisure facilities who previously took no physical exercise.
- Numbers of people incorporating physical activity into their everyday lifestyle.
- Uptake of sports and leisure services by particular target groups such as ethnic groups, youth, the unemployed, the mentally ill or the poor.

You will need to identify your performance indicators right from the start, and by monitoring them you will see whether you need to make any adjustments to the programme as you go along.

- *Self-evaluation* means asking yourself "What did I do well?" "What would I like to change?" and "How could I improve that next time?" All kinds of health promotion management can be subjected to this kind of process evaluation, whether it is planning and organizing the delivery of a health education programme or activity, facilitating the involvement of local groups in policy development and plans, organizing community-based work, developing and implementing policies, developing your staff or your organization, or working in partnership with other agencies. It is something you can do habitually, for example at the end of every day, or on completion of each particular task which contributes to your health promotion work.

- *Feedback from other people* is another way of evaluating performance. Giving and receiving feedback is an essential skill for all those involved in health promotion work, whether they are managers or front-line health promoters. Getting feedback from trusted colleagues on the health promotion work performance of your department, unit, team, service or business is a valuable form of peer evaluation. (I have already outlined some of the skills involved in Chapter 4. Techniques which improve effectiveness in giving feedback are also discussed in the section on "How to build health-promoting teams" in Chapter 7.) Staff should get regular feedback from their manager or team leader, and managers should ask for and get feedback from their staff, as part of the monitoring of the performance of a team or department.
- *Obtaining feedback from the clients or users themselves* should also be part of assessing the process of every intervention. The important thing is to encourage an atmosphere of openness and honesty, where problems can be confronted without people feeling blamed or judged as bad people. It can be done in many ways; simply *observing* clients and users accurately is an important tool. Do they look anxious or relaxed? Do they look interested and alert or bored and detached? You can also ask for feedback in various ways—through a suggestions box, through a "visitors book" inviting comments on a service, through a sensitive and accessible complaints procedure, through noting any spontaneous verbal feedback you receive or through asking questions.

Evaluating impact and measuring outcomes

Objectives are about changes you aim to make: changes in people's awareness, knowledge or behaviour, for example, or changes in policies, social and environmental conditions, or ways of working. Health promotion projects and programmes may also have objectives about changes in health status. So, for example, cardiac rehabilitation programmes may have the objective of reducing the numbers of patients who require further hospitalization. The following checklist indicates the kinds of changes you intend to make, and what methods you might use to assess or measure these changes.

Methods to evaluate changes in health awareness

- Measuring the interest shown by clients, students, service users or employees, for example how many people took up offers of leaflets, how many people enquired about preventive services.
- Monitoring changes in demand for health-related services.
- Analysis of media coverage.
- Questionnaires, interviews, discussion, observation with individuals or groups.

Methods to evaluate changes in knowledge, attitudes or empowerment

- Observing changes in what clients say and do: does this show a change in knowledge or attitudes or empowerment?
- Interviews and discussion involving question-and-answer between health promoter and clients
- Discussion and observation on how clients apply knowledge to real-life situations and how they solve problems.
- Use of attitude scales, self-esteem rating scales, or values-clarification tools.
- Observing how clients demonstrate their knowledge of newly acquired skills.
- Written tests, quizzes or questionnaires which require clients to answer questions about what they know. The results can be compared with tests undertaken before the health promotion activity or from a comparable group that has not received the health promotion.

Methods to evaluate behaviour change

- Observing what clients do.
- Recording behaviour. This could be records such as numbers attending a health promotion clinic or bringing their children to be vaccinated. Or it could be a periodical inventory, such as a follow-up questionnaire or interview to check on smoking habits six and 12 months after attending a stop-smoking group. Records of client behaviour can be compared with those of comparable groups in other areas, or with national average figures.

Methods to evaluate policy changes

- Policy statements and their implementation, such as increased introduction of "environmentally friendly" products in everyday use, or healthy eating choices in workplaces and schools.

continued on next page

continued

- Legislative changes, such as increased restriction on tobacco advertising.
- Changes in the availability of health-promoting products, facilities and services, such as low-cost recreational facilities or more health promotion clinics in primary health care settings or increases in the numbers of children's playgrounds in a locality.
- Changes in procedures or organization, such as more time being given to patient education.

Methods to evaluate changes in the physical and/or socio-economic environment

- Measuring physical changes such as levels of pollutants in the air.
- Measuring changes in the numbers of people living in overcrowded housing conditions.
- Measuring changes in the numbers of local people who are homeless.
- Measuring changes in the number of local people who are unemployed.

Methods to evaluate changes in health status

- Keeping records of health indicators such as weight, blood pressure, pulse rates on standard exercise, or cholesterol levels.
- Health surveys to identify larger-scale changes in health behaviour or health profiles of self-reported health outcomes.
- Analysis of trends in routine health statistics such as infant mortality rates or hospital admission rates.

There is a wide range of "off-the-shelf" measures available to assess changes in health status and much of the debate at present focuses on the relative merits of different measures in terms of their validity and reliability (14). But measurement tools may only be valid in the contexts for which they were designed, and will not necessarily be valid in other contexts. For example, a measure which is deemed to be valid for assessing health status in young people living in the USA will not necessarily be so in England. Given the complexity of choosing the best health outcomes measures, the Department of Health has commissioned the universities of Aberdeen and Leeds jointly to establish a UK Clearing House on Health Outcomes to collect, collate and disseminate the most up-to-date information on assessment of health outcomes (15). It is also available to provide expert advice on resource requirements, methodology, data collection systems, analysis and interpretation of health outcome studies.

In many instances it is not necessary or feasible to assess the long-term outcomes of a health promotion programme on health status. Evaluation of the more immediate effects may be more realistic. Nevertheless, it is important not to miss opportunities to identify indicators of health status. For example, cardiac rehabilitation programmes should be able to pick up any reduction in the numbers of patients being readmitted for treatment of cardiac problems. What will often be required to identify such indicators are closer links between health promotion programmes delivered in the community and the relevant hospital services.

Evaluation in practice: an evaluation of training on how to run preparation for parenthood classes in Powys (16)

The impetus for this work came from a multidisciplinary subgroup of the local Maternity Services Liaison Committee. A needs assessment exercise included surveying a sample of pregnant women, and this survey was carried out by lay representatives on the committee subgroup. As a result a pilot scheme to train teams of facilitators to run preparation for parenthood classes was commissioned. The team from each locality included a local health visitor, midwife and physiotherapist plus a lay representative and a health promotion specialist. The training involved training in team working, how to carry out groupwork with clients and training in evaluation methods. The evaluation of the training had several strands. The participants were interviewed before the training and several weeks later after they had the opportunity to deliver a preparation for parenthood programme in their locality. They also completed process evaluation questionnaires following each training day. Prior to the training most of the facilitators were not using evaluation methods with their preparation for parenthood classes, because of lack of time or lack of knowledge of methods. After the training all were using evaluation methods. Each team of facilitators evaluated their own preparation for parenthood classes. Of particular interest were responses from parents who had attended a class during an earlier pregnancy. This meant that comparisons could be made between the responses of those attending the classes run before and after the training. All but one of these prospective parents felt that the "new" classes had been better. Comments made included:

"Because we talked as a group and they (the facilitators) listened more."

"Made us feel part of the group—talked to rather than at."

The one woman who felt that the group had been the same still noticed the difference:

"The information was basically the same but the classes have been arranged differently and the members of the group have been encouraged to be more involved."

continued on next page

continued

After the pilot training over 100 health professionals were subsequently trained and the evaluations of the training were collated and included in a report to the Maternity Services Liaison Committee, so influencing the local health service purchaser's contract.

Anecdotal evidence of a "different cohort of clients who seem to be requiring less analgesia during childbirth and who are more in control of their birthing will need further research."

This evaluation therefore looked at three key levels at which judgements could be applied:

- The quality of the training itself (through process and outcomes evaluation of the training).
- The quality of the work activity of those trained (through process and impact evaluation of the outputs of the training, i.e. the preparation for parenthood classes).
- The quality of the outcomes of the activities of those trained (through assessing short-term outcomes via feedback from participants in the classes).

A range of evaluation methods were used, including questionnaires, group discussion and interviews. More long-term research will be required to make judgements about whether this training and the "new" classes have produced health benefits for the parents and/or their babies.

Review

The final stage of the health gain spiral is review. Whereas monitoring is an ongoing process, review is a method of taking stock at a particular point in the lifetime of a programme, project or service. This can involve taking a broad perspective on whether all the activities undertaken by a provider, or by a health alliance, or commissioned by a purchaser, are the best mix to attain the goals and objectives agreed and provide best value for money; or a particular manager could review whether a specific service needs redesigning to better match the resources available; or whether current provisions by a particular group of staff are still the most appropriate to meet changing needs. For example, imagine that you are the manager of a group of health visitors who run group sessions for parents of children under the age of five on home safety. Your monitoring shows that they spend most of their time discussing safe use of medicines and fire safety. You obtain and analyse the data from the local Accident and Emergency Department about the causes of accidents in children under five. These reveal that the major causes for admission of these children are road accidents and falls. You therefore decide to raise this with the health visitors in order to revise the home safety education. You also decide to join the local road safety alliance which includes membership from the local police and local authority, and to advocate that all local children's playgrounds have safety surfacing.

It is likely that major savings could be made on health service expenditure through improved health promotion. To take one example, the United Nations Children's Fund (UNICEF) argues that millions of pounds a year could be saved through the improved promotion of breast-feeding (17). It warns that breast-feeding is declining because hospitals are failing to support mothers adequately. In 1980 65% of mothers started breast-feeding. By 1990 only 63% began and a quarter gave up after six weeks. This is costing hospitals 12 times as much to treat gastrointestinal illnesses in bottle-fed babies, and in addition bottle-feeding is linked with other serious diseases such as childhood diabetes.

Health economics is one approach which is increasingly being used by commissioning agencies to assess whether efficient use is being made of scarce resources. Health economics is not simply concerned with saving money. It is primarily concerned with the relationship between costs and outcomes, and with making choices about what it is best to do. The health economist has a number of tools and concepts which can be used to help judgements to be made. For example, the concept of *opportunity cost* can be used to make judgements about which areas might best be invested in and what are areas for disinvestment. (Opportunity cost can be defined as the benefit which will be foregone by not investing in the best alternative use of resources.) The approaches of health economics have been criticized because of the difficulty of assigning costs to intangible aspects of well-being such as the relief of distress and worry. A detailed consideration of the contribution of health economics to health promotion is beyond the scope of this book, but further reading is suggested in the note at the end of the chapter (18).

An activity you could undertake: finding out about national and local health promotion strategies (19)

1. Have a look at the national strategy for health in your country (see note (2) at the end of this chapter). Try your local health promotion service if you do not have a copy.
2. What do you think are the good and not-so-good points about your national health strategy?
3. How does the health promotion work of your unit, service, department or business contribute to the aims set out in the national strategy?

continued on next page

continued

4. Find out if there is a local strategy for health in your district or locality. If so:
   - What do you think are the good and not-so-good points about your local health strategy?
   - How does your local strategy relate to your national strategy?
   - How does the health promotion work cf your unit, service, department or business contribute to the aims set out in the local strategy?

Questions you could ask yourself

Think about how you are evaluating one specific health promotion activity. Ask yourself the following questions:

1. Why are you evaluating it: which of the seven reasons you might have, described earlier in this chapter, apply? Can you identify any additional reasons?
2. To whom will the evaluation be made available? Have you specifically designed the evaluation to meet the needs of these people? If not, can you think of ways it could be improved?
3. Which evaluation methods are you using? Are these the most appropriate ones to tell you whether you are:
   - Monitoring performance and revising it on an ongoing basis?
   - Achieving your aims and objectives?
   - Identifying any unplanned spin-offs?
   - Identifying what to do next?

If not, what additional, or alternative, evaluation methods could you employ?

NOTES, REFERENCES AND FURTHER READING

(1) Explanation of terms often used when discussing planning and evaluation:

Control group: a comparison group, identified before a study is done, comprising persons who have not been exposed to an intervention, or other variable, the influence of which is being studied.

Cost effectiveness: cost effectiveness analysis is concerned with establishing the cost and effectiveness of an intervention in relation to a desired outcome. It could determine which set of activities requires the lowest cost input for a given outcome, or which produces the highest benefits (effectiveness) at a given cost level. In health promotion work, the outcomes may include many types of health gain, including extension of life expectancy or improved quality of life.

Evaluation: the process of critically assessing what has been achieved and how it has been achieved, related to a specific intervention.

Effectiveness what has been achieved, i.e. the outcomes in terms of benefits for an individual or a community. In health promotion work the outcomes are *health* benefits for an individual or community.

Efficacy: the extent to which an intervention produces a beneficial result under ideal conditions. Usually the determination of efficacy is based on the results of a randomized controlled trial.

Efficiency: how the outcome of an intervention has been achieved, i.e. how good (in terms of, for example, the relationship between inputs and outputs of resources), is the process. An efficient intervention is one that maximizes output for a given input, or minimizes input for a fixed output.

Health goal: a broad aspiration of an improved level of health which provides strategic direction for intervention.

Health indicator: a measure of health status or of a proxy factor associated with health status. Health indicators can be used to evaluate changes in the level of health of a population and, directly or indirectly, to assess the extent to which the objectives and targets of a programme are being attained.

Health objective: a specific, measurable level of health status for a defined population which will contribute to the achievement of a health goal. Health objectives provide yardsticks to assess progress towards health goals.

Health profiles: these provide measures of aspects of health so that assessment can be made of the effects of an intervention in terms of health gain (i.e., the outcomes on the health and well-being of the population concerned). For example, it is possible to measure subjective health status in different aspects of social functioning, for example physical mobility and the ability to perform specific tasks, such as make a cup of tea. On the basis of such studies it is possible to value health promotion and treatment interventions according to their positive impact on the health and well-being of people, rather than solely on their efficacy.

Health status: a measure of the overall health experience of an individual or a defined population.

Health target: a required improvement in health status by a given time which achieves a health objective.

Input: this is all the resources that go into a programme, service or activity, including money, time, staff, buildings and materials.

Instruments: in the context of health promotion work, this term denotes measuring devices, for example questionnaires, observation schedules, interview schedules.

Jarman index: a commonly used indicator of deprivation. The Jarman index was developed by analysing the answers that GPs gave to a series of questions which asked how much they considered 13 factors (such as the percentage of unemployment, percentage of living in overcrowded conditions and the number of households headed by someone born in the New Commonwealth or Pakistan) contributed to their workload. It was primarily a measure of the way in which certain social factors influence a GP's workload.

Objective: a specification of what it is intended to achieve through an intervention, i.e. the outcome.

Outcome: this is the end product of a programme or activity, expressed in appropriate terms of, for example, changes in people's attitudes, behaviour or knowledge, changes in health policy, changes in the uptake of services, changes in the rate of illness or accidents, changes in environmental conditions, or improvements to the health of the individuals, groups or communities concerned, as measured by outcome indicators.

Output the result of an activity, service or programme, in terms of the provision of facilities, services or procedures implemented, for example the services and facilities available to patients in a hospital ward.

Performance indicator: a defined measurable variable used to monitor the quality of management performance of an important aspect of health promotion work. Performance indicators may be activities (such as training events), resources (such as magazines or newsletters) or outcomes (such as numbers of accidents or sickness records) for which data are collected to allow comparison of performance for evaluation purposes.

Process what happens between input and outcome during an intervention, i.e. what the people involved do and how resources are used.

Qualitative: this is the term used to describe methods of assessment which express the outcome in words rather than numbers, and describe how good/bad the outcome was according to specified criteria. For example, an evaluation report of a screening programme for breast cancer might include users' descriptions of their experiences ("It was very painful"; "It was quick and well organized"; "It was embarrassing").

Quantitative: this is the term used to describe methods of assessment which are expressed in terms of numbers. For example, in the breast-screening evaluation, there could be an analysis that x number of women attended over period y, with an average throughput time of z minutes and $n\%$ called back for further tests. Often, both qualitative and quantitative descriptions and methods are used.

Randomized controlled trial: this involves making observations (or measurements) on a population which is then divided (by random sampling) into two equivalent groups: one of these is subjected to the intervention; after a predetermined time following the intervention, the observations are repeated and the results for the two groups are compared to establish whether or not the intervention had any effect.

Resource management: an approach to managing all resources (including money, staff, materials and buildings), which results in measurable improvements in health, through better-informed judgements about how the resources can be used to maximum effect. The four key elements contained within resource management related to health promotion work are:

- Improved quality of health promotion work.
- Involvement in management by all those staff such as doctors, nurses and the professions allied to medicine, whose decisions directly commit resources to health promotion activities.

- Improved information and communication.
- Effective control of use of resources.

See also the terms described in note (1) at the end of Chapter 4.

(2) The references for the four UK health strategies are provided in note (7) of Chapter 1. The reference for the Republic of Ireland strategy is provided in note (4) of this chapter.

The Health of the Nation strategy document has been followed by a *Health of the Nation* series of publications, including:

Department of Health (1993) *Key Area Handbooks* on:

CHD and Stroke
Cancers
Mental Illness
HIV/AIDS and Sexual Health
Accidents

These handbooks are available from BAPS, Health Publications Unit, Heywood Stores, Manchester Road, Heywood, Lancs OL10 2PZ.

First Steps for the NHS (1992): guidance to the NHS on how to start the process of implementing *The Health of the Nation.*

Working Together for Better Health (1993): a handbook of guidance on forming and operating alliances for health.

Local Target Setting: a discussion paper (1993): which discusses approaches to target setting below national level.

Ethnicity and Health: A guide for the NHS (1993): about applying *The Health of the Nation* strategy to ethnic groups.

Targeting Practice: The Contribution of Nurses, Midwives and Health Visitors to The Health of the Nation (1993).

One Year On: A Report on the Progress of The Health of the Nation (1993).

The Health of the Nation for Environmental Health (1993): published by the Institution of Environmental Health Officers (IEHO), Chadwick Court, 15 Hatfields, London, SE1 8DJ. Telephone: 0171 928 6006.

Targeting Practice: The Contribution of State Registered Dieticians to The Health of the Nation (1994).

Target is a quarterly *Health of the Nation* newsletter published by the Department of Health Strategy Unit.

These *Health of the Nation* publications are available from the Department of Health, Health Strategy Unit, Room LG04/05, Wellington House, 133–155 Waterloo Road, London SE1 8UG (Telephone: 0171 972 4466), apart from *The Health of the Nation for Environmental Health*, which is obtainable directly from the IEHO.

Nutrition and Health: A Management Handbook for the NHS (1994): This handbook, produced by the Nutrition Task Force (NTF), is available from the Health Publications Unit (BAPS, see address above).

Health Promoting Hospitals (1994): available from the Health Publications Unit (BAPS, see address above).

Health At Work in the NHS Action Pack (1992) London: Health Education Authority.

Health at Work in the NHS: Working Well—A Guide to Success (1994) London: Health Education Authority (a computerized resource and information pack).

Health of the Nation is published monthly as an insert to *NHS News* (the monthly newsletter published by the NHS Executive Communications Unit, available from NHS Executive Communications Unit, Department of Health, Room 8E39, Quarry House, Quarry Hill, Leeds LS2 7UE).

Other publications contain technical information on target setting, and survey data on public health:

Specification of National Indicators (1992).
Public Health Common Data Set (publications in 1992 and 1993).
Health Survey For England 1991 (1993).

(3) *Equality in health* is the absence in differences in health status among two or more population groups. Full equality in health may be impossible to achieve since some determinants cannot be controlled (for example sex, genetic factors). *Inequalities in health* are often caused by *inequities* (see notes on equity, below).

Equity in health is a moral value referring to justice and fairness, which is open to varying interpretations. It implies that ideally everyone should have a fair opportunity to attain his or her full health potential. Thus equity in health is concerned with creating equal opportunities for health and with bringing health differentials down to the lowest level possible.

Study after study has shown that socio-economic factors are among the most significant determinants of ill-health and there is convincing evidence of a widening of health inequalities between social groups in the UK in recent decades. For any age group, whether measuring mortality rates or different degrees of illness or disability, people in social group V (i.e., the poorest) come out worse than those in social groups I and II (i.e., the richest) by a factor of two or three. Many of those with the poorest health records and prospects are concentrated in particular neighbourhoods and estates. Action to improve the health of people living in these areas requires a wide range of health promotion programmes, which arguably should be given priority. See:

Townsend, P., Davidson, N and Whitehead, M. (1988) *Inequalities in Health.* Harmondsworth: Penguin.

More recent reports suggest that these inequalities are still widening. See:

Davey Smith, G., Bartley, M. and Blane, D. (1990) The Black Report on Socio-economic Inequalities in Health 10 years on. *British Medical Journal* **301**: 373–377.

Morris, J.N. (1990) Inequalities in Health: ten years and little further on. *Lancet*, 25 August: 491–493.

Whitehead, M. (1991) The concepts and principles of equity and health. *Health Promotion International*, **6**(3).

Jacobson, B., Smith, A. and Whitehead, M. (eds) (1991) *The Nation's Health: A Strategy for the 1990's*. (revised ed). King Edward's Hospital Fund for London. p. 114.

A study of health inequalities in the north of England (Cleveland, Cumbria, Durham, Northumberland and Tyne and Wear) over 10 years has found an "absolute" deterioration in health in the poorest areas; death rates among men under 45 and women over 65 have risen; and there has been an increase in the proportion of low-weight babies. See:

Department of Social Policy (1994) *Health and inequality: The Northern Region, 1981–91*. Newcastle upon Tyne: University of Newcastle upon Tyne.

A study over 10 years in Glasgow, between 1981 and 1991, shows that although overall death rates are falling, in the deprived areas of the city they fell at half the speed of the death rates in the richer parts of the city. Death rates have actually risen by 9% in the 15–44 year-old-age group in deprived areas. See:

McCarron, P., Davey Smith, G. and Womersley, J. (1994) Deprivation and Mortality in Glasgow: changes from 1980 to 1992. *British Medical Journal* **309** (6967): 1481.

For further information on deprivation and mortality in Scotland, see:

McLoone, P. and Boddy, F. (1994) Deprivation and mortality in Scotland 1981 and 1991. *British Medical Journal* **309** (6967): 1465.

A London School of Hygiene survey of 300 000 people in England showed poor people more likely to die before reaching 70, whether or not they lived in the more deprived areas. See:

Slogett, A. and Joshi, H. (1994) Higher mortality in deprived areas: personal or community disadvantage? *British Medical Journal* **309** (6967): 1470–1474.

A City University study confirmed a link between low birth weight and deprivation. The study of 17 000 babies born in Britain during one week in March 1958 showed those weighing under 61b at birth were likely to be more deprived during childhood and adolescence. See:

Bartley M., Power, C., Blane, D. *et al.* (1994) Birth weight and later socioeconomic disadvantage: evidence from the 1958 British cohort study. *British Medical Journal* **309** (6967): 1475–1478.

See also the editorials:

Davey Smith, G. and Morris, J. (1994) Increasing inequalities in the health of the nation. *British Medical Journal* **309** (6967): 1453.

Judge, K. (1994) Beyond health care. *British Medical Journal* **309** (6967): 1454.

Many experts would argue that the absence of safe, affordable housing for low-income families is a major contributor to ill-health. If people are living in overcrowded, unsafe, insanitary and poorly heated accommodation, disease and accidents inevitably follow. See:

Lowry, S. (1989) Housing and health: an Introduction to housing and health. *British Medical Journal* **299**: 1261–1262.

Lowry, S. (1989) Housing and health: temperature and humidity. *British Medical Journal* **299**: 1326–1328.

Lowry, S. (1989) Housing and health: indoor air quality. *British Medical Journal* **299**: 1388–1390.

Lowry, S. (1989) Housing and health: noise, space and light. *British Medical Journal* **299**: 1439–1442.

Lowry, S. (1990) Housing and health: health and homelessness. *British Medical Journal* **300**: 32–34.

Lowry, S. (1990) Housing and health: accidents at home. *British Medical Journal* **300**: 104–106.

Lowry, S. (1990) Housing and health: sanitation. *British Medical Journal* **300**: 177–179.

Lowry, S. (1990) Housing and health: families and flats. *British Medical Journal* **300**: 245–247.

Lowry, S. (1990) Housing and health: getting things done. *British Medical Journal* **300**: 390–392.

Shelter, (1989) *A Bad Start in Life: Children, Health and Housing*. London: Shelter.

It could therefore be argued that local authorities have a role which is at least as important as health authorities in commissioning the wide range of health promotion programmes (including housing and environmental improvement programmes) required to reduce inequalities in health.

Issues of race and health are another important aspect of work to reduce inequalities in health. Racism is institutionalized within our society and its organizations at every level. See:

Ahmad, W. (ed.) (1994) *"Race" and Health in Contemporary Britain.* Milton Keynes: Open University Press.

For further reading on health promotion for ethnic groups, see:

Department of Health (1993) *The Health of the Nation: Ethnicity and Health. A Guide for the NHS*. London: Department of Health.

Copies of this guide can be obtained by writing to Dr Andrew Clark, NHS Executive, Room 3W08, Quarry House, Quarry Hill, Leeds LS2 7UE.

One of the most recent contributions to the inequalities in the health debate is the report of the Commission on Social Justice (the Borrie report, commissioned by the Labour Party). This report argues that health policy should be reorientated towards health promotion with the aim of improving health and reducing health inequalities. It identifies four factors which affect people's health that can be influenced by public policy: individual lifestyle, social and community networks, living and working conditions, and social, economic and environmental circumstances. See:

Miliband, D. (ed.) (1994) *Social Justice: Strategies for National Renewal. The Report of the Commission on Social Justice*. London: Institute of Public Policy Research/Vintage.

(4) Parston, G. (1994) Eire health policy: power with responsibility. *Health Service Journal* **104** (5426): 25.

See also the Eire health strategy document:

Department of Health (1994) *Shaping a Healthier Future*. Dublin: Stationery Office.

The Republic of Ireland's new health strategy document is available from Government Publications Office, Sun Alliance House, Molesworth Street, Dublin 2, Eire.

(5) Huxham, C. and Macdonald, D. (1992) Introducing collaborative advantage: achieving inter-organizational effectiveness through meta-strategy. *Management Decision* **30** (3): 50–56.

(6) This case study is based on:

Standish, S., Perry, C. and Palk, N. (1994) Joint commissioning: scoring doubles. *Health Service Journal* **104** (5420): 26–27.

(7) This section is partly based on a discussion on objectives and targets in:

Ewles, L. and Simnett, I. (3rd edn, 1995) *Promoting Health: A Practical Guide*. London: Scutari Press. Ch. 6.

(8) For an example of a mission statement see Chapter 3.

(9) Glaxo (1993) *Setting Targets as Part of the Health Gain Cycle*. Uxbridge, Middlesex: Glaxo Pharmaceuticals Ltd.

For open learning material on targets, see the unit "Objectives and Targets for Health Gain" (written by Ina Simnett) in the volume *Needs Assessment for Health Improvement and Health Gain*, which is part of the *Managing Health Improvement Project* (MAHIP) material. For information about the availability of these materials, see note (8) in Chapter 1.

(10) This section is partly based on information in:

Ewles, L. and Simnett, I. (3rd edn, 1995) *Promoting Health: A Practical Guide*. London: Scutari Press. Ch. 6.

(11) For further reading on evaluation, see:

Downie, R.S., Fyfe, C. and Tannahill, A. (1990) *Health Promotion: Models and Values*. Oxford: Oxford University Press. Ch. 5.

Whitehead, M. and Tones, K. (1991) *Avoiding the Pitfalls*. London: Health Education Authority.

Grassle L. and Kingsley S. (1986) *Measuring Change, Making Changes: An Approach to Evaluation*. London: National Community Health Resource.

Feuerstein M. (1986) *Partners in Evaluation: Evaluating Development and Community Programmes with Participants*. London: Macmillan.

Tones K., and Tilford S. (2nd edn, 1994) *Health Education: Effectiveness, Efficiency and Equity*. London: Chapman & Hall.

Nutbeam, D., Smith, C. and Catford J. (1990) Evaluation in health education: a review of progress, possibilities and problems. *Journal of Epidemiology and Community Health* **44**: 83–89.

Tolley K. (1993) *Health Promotion: How to Measure Cost-effectiveness*. London: Health Education Authority.

For open learning material on evaluation, see the unit on "Planning and Delivering Quality Health Promotion Work" in the volume *Quality Issues in Health Promotion Work*, which is part of the *Managing Health Improvement Project* (MAHIP) material. For information about the availability of these materials, see note (8) in Chapter 1.

Examples of evaluated programmes which include useful discussions of the evaluation process are:

Pye M. and Kapila M. (1990) *AIDS Programme: Evaluation of AIDS Health Promotion Programmes*. AIDS Programme Paper Number 7. London: Health Education Authority.

Stewart-Brown S.L. and Prothero D.L. (1988) Evaluation in community development. *Health Education Journal* **47** (4).

For a comprehensive text on health promotion planning, including evaluation, see:

Green, L. and Kreuter, M. (2nd edn, 1991) *Health Promotion Planning*. Toronto: Mayfield.

(12) These indicators were developed for Health at Work in the NHS in Wessex. See:

Wessex Institute of Public Health Medicine (1994) *Indicators and Outcome Measures for Health at Work in the NHS in Wessex*. Available from Annette Rushmere, Health Promotion Manager, Wessex Institute of Public health Medicine, Dawn House, Highcroft, Romsey Road, Winchester S022 5DH. Telephone: 01962 863511.

(13) This is adapted from information in a computerized resource pack:

Health Education Authority (1994) *Working Well: A Guide to Success*. London: HEA/NHS Executive.

(14) Harries, U. and Hill, S (1994) Measuring outcomes: two sides of the coin. *Health Service Journal* **104** (5421): 25.

(15) UK Clearing House for Information on the Assessment of Health Outcomes, Nuffield Institute for Health Service Studies, 71–75 Clarendon Road, Leeds, LS2 9PL. Telephone: 01532 45034.

(16) This case study is based on an evaluation report, available from Ffion Lloyd-Williams, Health Promotion Unit, Mansion House, Bronllys, Powys LD3 OLS. Telephone: 01874 711661.

(17) Reported by James Erlichman in *The Guardian*, 23 November 1994, p. 9.

(18) For a more detailed discussion of health economics, see the unit "Setting Priorities for Health Gain" (written by Peter Brambleby), in the volume *Needs Assessment for Health Improvement and Health Gain*, which is part of the *Managing Health Improvement Project* (MAHIP) open learning material. For information about the availability of these materials, see note (8) in Chapter 1.

See also:

Donaldson, C. and Mooney, G. (1991) Needs assessment, priority setting and contracts for health care: an economic view. *British Medical Journal* **303**: 1029–1030.

Mooney, G., Gerard, K., Donaldson, C. and Farrar, S. (1992) *Priority Setting in Purchasing: Some Practical Guidelines*. Research Paper 6. Birmingham: National Association of Health Authorities and Trusts.

Maynard, A. (1991) The relevance of health economics to health promotion. In Badura, B. and Kickbusch, I. (eds), *Health Promotion Research: Towards a New Social Epidemiology*. Copenhagen: WHO Regional Publications. European Series No. 37.

(19) This activity is based on an activity in Ewles, L. and Simnett, I. (3rd edn, 1995) *Promoting Health: a Practical Guide*. London: Scutari Press. Ch. 6. It is reproduced with kind permission from Scutari Press.

CHAPTER 7 Improving management processes for health development

Summary

The chapter focuses on some of the critical competencies you will need in order to manage effectively for health gain: the ability to lead health development; the ability to use new management thinking; the ability to facilitate (enable) others to do things rather than doing them yourself; the ability to resolve conflicts and improve the quality of working life; the ability to build autonomous teams capable of creatively moving forward in health development in turbulent times; and the ability to work collaboratively, in health alliances, with other agents and agencies who may have very different views and ways of working to your own. An activity you could undertake to assess your leadership potential, and some questions you could ask yourself, complete the chapter.

"It's not just what you do, but the way that you do it."

In this chapter I focus on the way you manage in order to achieve better health, and at the heart of this lies your understanding of, and relationships with, other people. These are aspects of your work which you are not often asked to report on. But these implicit aspects of your health promotion management work are the key to success. I start by looking at what is a core competency for the management of health promotion: leadership.

SPREADING LEADERSHIP

As we have seen, developing health-promoting organizations and communities will involve rethinking and reshaping the role of organizations. This will require all those involved in the management of health promotion to take an enhanced leadership role. For example, health promotion is at the heart of the work of the new health authorities and health commissions. They must assume leadership of the local health agenda, building and sustaining coalitions for health gain with all relevant parties. In the management of health promotion, they will need to be much more active in health lobbying and campaigning, advocating real change to improve the health of local communities. A more assertive and high-profile stance will also be required from all those working as providers of health promotion. We shall need to *spread* leadership, not just vest it in those with high status in organizations.

The leadership vacuum in the NHS has been pointed out by some of the top health management experts, including Peter Griffiths, director of the King's Fund College (1). It has been argued that the NHS reforms have divided people into the "doers" and the "done-to" (2). The doers include ministers, senior managers, clinical directors, authority and board members, GP fundholders and commissioners. The done-to include non-purchasing GPs, middle managers, junior doctors, nurses, the professions allied to medicine, administrative and clerical staff, ancillary staff and patients. On the whole, power, influence and budgets are vested in the doers, who have welcomed the challenge of the reforms. The done-to are relatively powerless and can feel vulnerable, out of control and fearful. The sort of leaders required in this situation are enthusiastic doers who have the ability to change those who are done-to into doers, i.e. to develop others as leaders.

This suggests that the sort of leaders needed are those who (3):

- Can boost morale.
- Can be there for bad times as well as good.
- Will be prepared to stay for a long time (at least several years).
- Will breed other leaders.
- Are capable of spreading a strategic vision.

British health care has traditionally separated much of the responsibility for management from the clinical and health promotion roles carried out by the health professions. While there is obviously a need for some professional managers and focused clinicians/health promoters, the notion that these should be distinct is incompatible with the delivery of high-quality, cost-effective services (4). This is especially true of the management and leadership of health promotion, which requires an integrated approach across all managers and health professions. The attributes needed to reinvent organizations such as hospitals as health-promoting ones are not just good managerial skills but the ability to lead.

The attributes of good leaders

Good leaders are inspirational. It is to such leadership that sport owes much of its importance as an integral part of our lives. Without it, most sporting contests would simply be won by the strongest or the most skilful. The great sports coaches, by teaching athletes not to be over-awed by superior forces and galvanizing the most unlikely material into winning units, not only make sport itself more dramatic but inspire all of us to make more of our own potential. What is the secret of leaders like Sir Matt Busby? Above all they are good motivators. But there are many different ways to motivate, such as appealing to the emotions, or the ability to bring the best out in people. Perhaps the most successful leaders have three key attributes:

- They know themselves well enough to use the approach most appropriate to themselves.
- They know their teams well enough to use the approach most appropriate to the people concerned.
- They know their field of expertise well enough to use the best approach for the circumstances.

In other words, good leaders have good judgement: of themselves, of their chosen sphere of expertise and of those they are leading.

There is no easy way to become a good leader. The following pointers may help:

Pointers towards good leadership

1. *Be humble and tolerant*: the most effective leaders are often those who are not too proud to admit their faults, admit to being wrong, listen to the criticisms of others and are open to new ideas.
2. *Listen*: effective leaders are good listeners. They try to understand the other person's position. This increases their chances of making the right decisions and successfully communicating their views or influencing others.
3. *Think*: few of us use more than a small fraction of our mental powers while we are working. Half an hour spent simply reflecting on a project before you start can save weeks (or months) of unproductive effort later on. It is also vital to improve the quality of thinking, and some suggestions were made in Chapter 2 about how to do this.
4. *Inform*: get people together, tell them what's going on, what you are trying to do and why.
5. *Develop people*: if you just bemoan the fact that people to whom you might delegate are not up to it, you will always have problems making

continued on next page

continued

things any better. Invest time and effort in training, supporting and encouraging others (consider their needs for personal development, professional development and managerial development) and in the long run everyone will gain.

6. *Trust*: give people freedom to use their initiative. The most effective work is often done by teams committed to group objectives. If you wish to produce such work you must learn to see yourself as a team leader who is also a team member. Trust is then based on genuine engagement with the team.
7. *Build teams*: all leaders are team builders because teams are always improving or declining in their performance. Therefore the work of team building is never done.

The leader is a teacher

Leaders do a lot of teaching—such as giving instructions, coaching, and explaining new policies and procedures. Yet they often don't receive training in how to carry out this important function. Teaching people effectively is a very complex activity, partly because learning requires change and is mentally and emotionally hard work, and often because many people have felt "put down" in school by their teachers. This means that when leaders teach they must avoid, above all, making their staff feel they are "being treated like children".

Imagine that a member of your staff responds to teaching with comments such as:

"I've always done it this way."
"What's wrong with doing it like this?"
"I don't get it."
"I can't do it that way."

Your staff member has encountered a barrier to learning, and you must stop teaching and help her or him to work through this barrier through *listening*.

To take another example, a surprising amount of teaching assumes that it is the teacher who is more active—telling, explaining, presenting—and the learner who is more passive. Yet we know from research that much more learning occurs when this is reversed—when the learner is more active. Getting learners more actively involved and participating in the learning process is the mark of an effective teacher. To do this you must *help learners to talk* (5).

There is also evidence (6) that learning can be improved by making learners more aware of their habitual learning styles. This may be because they are then able to build on their strengths (the learning styles they are most comfortable with) but also, through awareness of the learning styles they are least likely to use, learners can consciously practise these alternative ways of learning and build a more flexible learning repertoire (i.e. a stock of regularly used techniques).

There are two key dimensions concerned with how people learn (7), which operate independently:

1. *The holistic versus analytic dimension*: people who prefer to use the analytical style are analytic, deductive, rigorous and critical. They tend to think things through step by step in an objective analytical way. People who habitually prefer to use the holistic style can be described by words such as synthetic, inductive, divergent and creative. They may be impatient with much reflection, and like to try things out in an unstructured way.
2. *The verbalizer versus the imager*: verbalizers are inclined to represent information verbally when they are thinking while imagers represent it in the form of mental images. Imagers learn best from pictorial presentations, verbalizers from verbal presentations. Imagers recall highly descriptive text better than complex and unfamiliar text, while the reverse is true for verbalizers.

Through helping learners to identify their own habitual learning styles, the teacher can help learners to be more flexible and adaptable through encouraging them to use non-preferred styles. This has the advantage of actively involving learners in restructuring the information and concepts to be learned, and so itself leads to better learning. In other words, teachers must focus on the process of learning (helping people to learn how to learn) as well as the content.

In summary, there is no one "best" way to learn, but using a wide variety of ways can help people to learn effectively in a range of different situations. Further reading is suggested in the note at the end of the chapter (8).

Finally:

> Goodness in the moral sense is the sure foundation of leadership.
>
> John Adair

FACILITATION

In the final analysis, in the process of managing you are totally dependent on other people, and your effectiveness is limited or enhanced by their qualities, abilities and motivation. How effective you are at getting the best out of other people will depend not only on your skills but also on your attitudes. Your attitudes and values have a very significant influence on your "human skills" (these are often alternatively called "life skills"). You may regard yourself as having very balanced attitudes and values which never cause any problem except when you are faced with biased people and extremists. This is a false assumption. We are all biased in one direction or another. The truly unprejudiced person does not exist.

So your attitudes will influence your effectiveness as a manager. The problem, of course, is that there are no "right" attitudes—only appropriate attitudes or inappropriate attitudes for the particular circumstances. In order to get the best out of others, it is essential for you to develop your ability to see matters from a range of viewpoints, and to do this you will need to challenge your existing attitudes and values at every opportunity! To do this will require you to identify your own attitudes and to question whether they are the appropriate attitudes for your circumstances at work.

How to facilitate

Facilitation has a key part to play in the promotion and improvement of health. Thus, for example, the new health authorities will be responsible not so much for developing their own health strategies, but for enabling the development of agreed local health gain strategies which are owned by all local agencies and people. This is an important shift of emphasis, because increasingly it will be GPs and local authorities, schools and other agencies who actually purchase the interventions and services to implement the health strategies. As authority and responsibility are increasingly devolved from commissioners to purchasers and from purchasers to providers, enabling others, rather than doing it yourself, will be a key function of many local organizations and thus their staff.

I shall illustrate how to set about facilitating someone to do something through looking at delegation. Delegation is one of the most difficult aspects of managing. It means giving someone else the *authority* (and the resources and time) to do something on your behalf. You retain *responsibility* for it and you must therefore have some form of control in order to ensure that the required results are achieved. Even experienced managers can have qualms about this. These qualms often stem from fears that the person doing the task might not do it the "right" way (i.e. the manager's way!). This short-sighted view fails to distinguish between obtaining the required results and obtaining them in a particular way. Facilitation is about giving people the freedom to do things their own way. So a facilitative approach to delegating a task would be to:

1. Agree with the person to whom you are delegating the task what is to be achieved (i.e. the objectives and targets).
2. Agree the best methods for measuring how well the task is done and how successful are the outcomes (i.e. methods for evaluation of process and outcomes).
3. Agree how progress will be checked on (i.e. monitoring methods).
4. Agree a review date, to provide feedback, support, guidance and coaching, if necessary, or to identify how the person can be delegated further tasks, in order to improve competencies or take on new roles, if appropriate.

Facilitation is thus no easy option. It is not about being permissive (letting people go their own way); it is a highly skilled way of empowering others and involves continuously developing and supporting them. Well done, it is a good investment for individuals, and for better health-promoting management of organizations.

DEVELOPING NEW MANAGEMENT

I have already discussed, in Chapter 2, "new management" thinking. The organizations of the late 1990s and 2000s will mainly be a network of "semi-autonomous teams"—independent, flexible and highly trained. One of the easiest ways to understand the difference between "old-style" organizations and the new, "organic" organizations is to contrast the BBC with Channel 4. The BBC was at its height in the 1960s. It had a Board of Governors, Board of Management, Programme Directorate, Finance Directorate, and huge departments which all employed many full-time staff working exclusively for the BBC. Channel 4 has a small central organization planning the schedules and commissioning or acquiring programmes, and is supplied by a network of relatively small facilities and freelancers, all of whom are free to prospect for new opportunities and experiment with new products. As Eastern Europe shows, the break-up of the paralysing rigidity of an omnipotent central authority brings dangers of chaos. One of the main difficulties in instituting the new order is in changing the attitudes and behaviour of those who were brought up under the old system. The changes required are summarized in the following box.

Old management into new management

Old managers saw themselves as a link in the chain of command.	New managers see their chief job as the leader of a team.
Old managers saw their chief job as giving directions to employees.	New managers see their chief job as getting ideas from the team.
Old managers allocated the performance of tasks.	New managers communicate an understanding of objectives and empower people to solve problems.
The old manager's chief concern was to satisfy corporate objectives.	The new manager's chief concern is to understand and satisfy customer needs.
The old manager saw training as the responsibility of the personnel department.	The new manager sees the development of people as his or her own responsibility, met by talking to people, learning together and training.
The old managers saw other departments and organizations as rivals.	The new manager sees them as allies in the quest to meet customer needs.

These are differences in attitude, which are not confined to those with the title of manager, but are equally found in all professions and occupations. How do these attitudes show themselves in practice? Look for the following if you want to examine your own behaviour for signs of "old management thinking". The old manager:

- Spends too much time in the office dealing with paper and too little time dealing with people.
- Deals with staff individually in his or her office rather than as a group.
- Imposes his or her ways of working and system of organization on the team without discussion.
- Sees other groups and organizations as rivals and takes a defensive attitude towards them.
- Insists on all decisions being cleared with himself or herself.
- Finds solutions to problems on his or her own, without asking the team for their ideas.
- Gets people trained only to the level necessary to perform the job. Sees no point in developing the capabilities of staff beyond the immediate needs of the tasks they are currently required to perform.
- Never reviews performance with the team, and takes any suggestion that things could have been done better as personal criticism.

If you recognize any of these habits in yourself, try to develop the seven pointers of a good leader, set out in the section on "Spreading leadership". Further reading is suggested in the note at the end of the chapter (9).

HOW TO RESOLVE CONFLICTS AND IMPROVE THE QUALITY OF WORKING LIFE

Conflicts are inevitable in human relationships, and are especially frequent in organizations which are developing and changing. They often surface when teams are trying to finalize decisions as part of the problem-solving process. So, although some conflicts can be prevented by good and open communication, it is essential for leaders to understand and use effective approaches to resolve conflicts. There are three basic ways to deal with conflict (10). Two are ineffective, and only the third way is effective. Unfortunately, most of us have experienced only the first two ways and do not realize that there is another alternative. The ineffective ways are *win/* lose methods of conflict resolution. They both result in someone winning and the other person losing.

- Method 1: I win–you lose (authoritarian conflict resolution).
- Method 2: you win–I lose (*laissez-faire*, permissive, conflict resolution).

Through using the third method no one loses, so it has been called the "no-lose" method or the "win–win" method. Acquiring a high level of competence with this method is not easy—it requires a lot of practice. It requires leaders to use assertive skills and listening skills in an integrated way. To use the no-lose method you need to:

1. Stop sending judgemental or blaming *you* messages, such as:

   "*You* shouldn't do that."
   "*You* should know better."
   "Why don't *you* ..."
   "*You* ought to ..."

   Instead send assertive *I* messages, such as:

   "*I'm* upset about this because we won't meet the deadline."
   "*I* am worried about these incomplete forms because our records on the project are not accurate."

   When you send *I* messages you appeal for help, and own that you have a problem. This is more effective than demands, threats or lectures. A common response to *I* messages is for the receiver to become defensive, upset or resistive. To deal with this you need to "shift gear" and to:

2. *Listen*, and reflect back the feelings, defences and reasons of the other person, because it communicates your understanding and acceptance of the other person's feelings and position. So you might say:

   "You were so short of time, you felt you couldn't take the time to fill in the forms?"

3. *Clarify the problem*: through listening you will be able to identify the underlying problem, or the blockage which is causing the presenting problem, and through clarifying the real problem it may be possible for you together to identify a solution which meets the needs of both parties. (For more information on problem solving, see the section on "How to work together for better health" later in this chapter.)

Using the no-lose method means that you respect the needs of the other person, but you are nevertheless persistent in your search for a solution which meets your own needs. It builds mutual trust, respect and openness. For further reading on conflict resolution, see the suggestions in the note at the end of the chapter (11).

Nationally, the Advisory, Conciliation and Arbitration Service (ACAS) is an independent statutory body responsible for promoting good relationships between employers, employees and their representatives. As part of this function, it aims to improve the quality of working life for people at all levels in organizations and at the same time produce benefits in terms of the operational effectiveness of organizations (12). From the observations of ACAS some of the worst workplace stressors include:

- Insecurity or fear of redundancy.
- Autocratic management styles which are demotivating and in the extreme are nothing less than "bullying".
- Erratic or inconsistent management strategies.
- Poor working conditions.
- Lack of opportunity to influence the way work is carried out—and the under-valuing of the employee's skill and talent.
- Poor communication processes—often only one way (top-down) and with little feedback of employees' views.

To tackle these issues ACAS recommends a Quality of Working Life (QWL) strategy. The main strands of a QWL strategy are:

- People will be better motivated if the work experience satisfies their social and psychological needs in addition to economic needs.

- Individual motivation and therefore greater efficiency can be enhanced by attention to the design of jobs and work organization.
- People work more effectively if they are managed in a participative way.

QWL echoes many of the features of health-promoting organizations, which I first set out in Chapter 1, and which have formed a thread throughout this book. QWL recognizes that managers and employee representatives have a joint interest in creating organizations that meet both business and human needs. QWL organizations include many or most of the following features:

- A statement of organization philosophy and values.
- A "participative" management style.
- A flat organizational structure.
- QWL-based job design.
- Effective communications.
- Joint problem solving.
- Reward strategies focusing on the organization, the team and skill acquisition (rather than on individual performance-related pay).
- Selection processes emphasizing individual attitudes and personal characteristics.
- A continuous process of training.
- "Developmental" performance appraisal.

QWL job design principles

Ideally jobs should:

- Form a coherent whole, so that performance of the job makes a significant contribution to the outcomes of the intervention or service.
- Provide some variety of method, location or skill.
- Allow for some discretion and employee control in the way the work is done.
- Include some responsibility for outcomes.
- Provide opportunity for learning and problem solving.
- Be seen as leading towards some form of desirable future.
- Provide opportunity for development in ways the individual finds relevant.

In summary, QWL approaches embody mentally, emotionally and socially "healthy" workplace policies and practices, and thus contribute to the primary prevention of mental illness created through workplace stressors

(13). As such they have a key part to play in health-promoting organizations. For further discussion on how to promote health at work, see Chapter 8.

HOW TO BUILD HEALTH-PROMOTING TEAMS

Research shows that healthy families have "an affiliative attitude" (14). They are not only warm, affectionate and supportive to family members, but reach out to neighbours and are valued members of their communities. This capacity for closeness and involvement is nevertheless accompanied by respect for individual differences. The same is true of successful organizations and teams: an affiliative attitude prevails towards customers, employees, and other organizations and people with whom they work in partnership. As in healthy families, such teams and organizations are guided by principles which transcend profit motives. Many explicitly base their philosophy on religious values. More important, though, than adherence to a particular creed, is adherence to ethical principles which are shared by many of the religions and moral philosophies. These include a positive view of what people are capable of if they are trusted, motivated and provided with good working conditions, and a belief that honesty, giving good value and providing good service are all worthwhile things in themselves. Just as healthy families foster autonomy and individuality, so successful organizations and teams encourage independence and delegation. Large organizations are divided into small teams (ideally with 7–12 members) in which healthy family-type interactions are possible. Two opposing characteristics are shown by healthy organizations: opportunities for freedom and innovation by the teams, combined with the discipline and control created by the central body (such as the board of directors) through a clear sense of purpose, shared values and an agreed strategy.

There are three key characteristics of effective teams:

1. A clear, agreed objective.
2. Agreed roles for each member of the team.
3. Trust between team members.

There are two quite distinct types of role which team members can adopt, and a team will only function with maximum effectiveness if everyone knows their role in both senses. First there is the "expert role": the expertise each member brings to the team, such as expertise in research and evaluation, in marketing and working with the mass media, in community-based work or in financial management. Second there are "functional roles" which are concerned not with what is done, but how it is done. For a team to achieve synergy (a team in which the whole is greater than the sum of the parts) it has to achieve appropriate allocation of these functional roles—so that, for example, there are not two people trying to be leaders. This is an area in which the work of Dr Meredith Belbin has been extremely influential (15). By giving names to and describing these roles, he assisted communication and enabled effective team development. He identified these "archetypal" functional roles through observing the working of hundreds of teams. Thus, according to Belbin, an ideal team contains one of each of the following.

Functional roles in teams

- *Plant*: creative, imaginative, unorthodox. The creative source of ideas to solve difficult problems. (Weakness: can be bad at communicating with "ordinary" people.)
- *Coordinator*: mature, confident, trusting. A good leader or chairperson. Clarifies goals and promotes decisions. (Not necessarily the most intelligent member of the team.)
- *Shaper*: dynamic, outgoing, highly strung. Challenges, pressurizes, encourages the team to get on with its tasks. (Might be seen as aggressive or prone to bursts of temper.)
- *Teamworker*: social, mild, perceptive, accommodating. Listens and supports members of the team. (Indecisive in crunch situations, compromises to avoid conflict.)
- *Completer*: painstaking, conscientious, anxious. Searches out errors, ensures that the team completes its work on time. (May worry unduly, may be reluctant to delegate.)
- *Implementer*: disciplined, reliable, conservative, efficient. Turns ideas into actions. Good at organizing. (May be inflexible.)
- *Resource investigator*: extrovert, enthusiastic, communicative. Good at networking with other people and agencies. (May lose interest after initial enthusiasm.)
- *Specialist*: single-minded, dedicated. Brings knowledge or skills in rare supply. (Contributes only on a narrow front.)
- *Monitor/evaluator*: critical, strategic, discerning. Analyses options, makes judgements. (Lacks ability to inspire others.)

Thinking about these categories of team roles can help you to identify functional problems in teams you work in, and give you ideas about how these problems could be solved. It can also help you to modify your own teamworking approach and to contribute better (Belbin found that people who do not fit into one of these nine categories tend not to contribute much to the teams they are in) (16). The better balanced a team is in terms of these functional roles, the easier it is for it to move towards the third prerequisite for synergy: trust. Once members of a team understand how they can best contribute to the team, in terms of their roles, and know that they are valued for their unique contributions, then they no longer need to compete against each other. Then they can perform to their maximum ability, and the whole will become more than the sum of its parts.

How teams can learn to trust each other

The first step in team building is to help members to become aware of what they do and how others respond. This means that teams must develop the ability to give each other feedback in a straightforward, descriptive way, rather than in a judgemental or critical way. Then, members are able to take in the feedback, while retaining self-awareness and self-confidence, and to evaluate whether, and how, they need to change. This involves avoiding doing some of the things which are almost "second nature", and instead substituting helpful processes which nurture respect and trust. The things team members need to *stop* doing are:

- Giving other members advice.
- Telling other members what to do.
- Expressing judgements or opinions about the personal characteristics or behaviour of other members or about the team.

Techniques for helping teams to give each other constructive and descriptive feedback are set out in the following box.

Giving feedback in teams

At each team meeting set aside time for the following activities. Ensure that team members are sitting in a circle, and that each member has a clear view of all other members, for these activities. Undertake these activities in the sequence set out below.

1. First ask each team member, in turn, to report back on *what they have noticed*, since the previous meeting, related to how the work of the team is being carried out. Each member should have the opportunity, without interruption or discussion, to say what they remember seeing or hearing during performing team tasks.
2. Second, complete a round of statements, by each team member in turn, on *what each member has felt* about the work of the team since the previous meeting (again without interruptions, comments or discussion).

continued on next page

continued

3. Third, complete a round of statements in answer to the following question: *What, if anything, do you want to change*? If a team member is addressing a request for change to one other individual, the two people concerned should look each other directly in the eye.
   It may help if someone volunteers to act as "scribe" and writes up all the responses to each round on separate sheets of flip-chart paper, which can then be "posted" on the walls, and assist the processes of discovery and learning.
   A further deepening of awareness may also come by team members challenging statements which they feel are opinions rather than descriptions (for example, "I felt that we did well" is an opinion; "I felt pleased" is a feeling. "I noticed that we were better organized" is an opinion; what you might have noticed could be: "I noticed that we made an agenda at the beginning of this meeting").
4. Finally, complete a round of statements, by each team member in turn, in answer to the following question: *What actions, if any, do you now intend to take*?

It will feel uncomfortable, at first, completing this sequence, but the more this safe, enabling structure is used, the more open feedback will become, and the more trust and respect will develop.

As it becomes established as a team norm that members can report what they observe happening, what they feel, what they need to work effectively, and what actions they will take to work together more effectively, so synergy will begin to operate, and the team will begin to generate ideas about how to improve performance which none of the members could have had on their own. There are many other activities which can be undertaken to enhance team performance, and some suggestions for further study are provided at the end of the chapter (17). The most important point to note is that learning to trust each other is a process, not a one-off event, and that teams must actively work on this process, as well as on their objectives and tasks, in order to become effective.

Understanding team development

Teams have their own "life cycles" and tend to show particular patterns of behaviour at each stage in their life cycle. This cycle has been categorized as having five stages and the behaviour patterns which characterize each stage are (18):

1. *Forming*: this team is in the process of forming and needs time to establish its ground rules, clarify its purpose and help members to

identify their roles. If this fails to happen, the team could fail to progress to the next stage in the development cycle, and will be stuck with unclear objectives, weaknesses covered up, inability to generate ideas, poor listening, members' feelings not expressed or dealt with, and the leader making most of the decisions.

2. *Storming*: this stage begins when members decide to do something about improving the performance of the team. The team begins to experiment, face problems more openly and consider a wider range of options before making decisions. The leader may be challenged and members may get into heated discussions about how things are done. For the first time the members of the team begin to understand each other and show more concern for the views and problems of each other. This can be a difficult period for everyone, but it is a vital stage in the team's maturing process, rather like the period of rebelling and questioning in adolescence.
3. *Norming*: successful handling of the storming stage leads to the development of open communication and trust. The team now has the confidence to examine its working methods and to agree rules and procedures which everyone contributes to framing and to which everyone is committed.
4. *Performing*: the team is now mature and is characterized by flexibility, trust, openness, honesty, cooperation and confrontation. A continual review of performance and results becomes part of a way of life.
5. *Ending*: many teams have a limited time-span, meeting until a particular task has been completed. At the end of a team's life, it is natural for members to feel a sense of loss. It may be helpful to have a final "rounding-up" session, which could give team members an opportunity to express their appreciation of each other, their sadness at parting, and perhaps arrange a follow-up or "reunion".

When a team fails to mature in some way, sabotage attempts may occur. It is thus essential for teams to invest time and effort on the process of development, and to diagnose and deal with any blocks which prevent them reaching the stage of performing to full capacity.

What makes teams inventive?

One recent study tried to isolate the most important factors in determining whether a team was innovative (19). The most significant predictors were creativity of team members, the climate of the team and the length of time they had worked together. Four factors in the overall climate of a team together predicted the innovativeness of the team:

- A clear set of objectives.
- High levels of participation.
- Task orientation.
- Support for innovation.

The authors of this study concluded that to be innovative teams should ensure that they have:

- Selected creative members.
- Clear and agreed objectives.
- High levels of information sharing.
- Involvement of team members in decision making.
- High levels of interaction between members.
- High quality of decision making through constructive controversy and critical self-appraisal.
- Active support to the team for innovation through providing them with cooperation, time and resources for innovation.

The best predictor of the likely effectiveness of innovations introduced by teams was the length of time members had worked together. The longer a team had been together, the more effective were changes they introduced likely to be perceived (however, most of the teams studied had been together for less than two years, and this study does not show whether the performance of teams, on criteria of effectiveness of innovations, may be adversely affected by working together for an extremely long time). Nevertheless, it suggests that to get the best (most effective) innovations out of teams it is desirable to build them and maintain them in a relatively stable form for at least two to three years.

HOW TO WORK IN PARTNERSHIPS FOR BETTER HEALTH

Developing joint local health strategies which are owned and shared by many different local agencies and people, and involve complex networks of people working together for better health, is a big challenge. Negotiations can be lengthy, particularly when a shared local health strategy is being entered into for the first time, or when a number of agencies are planning to work together for the first time. It is therefore essential for all those concerned to allocate plenty of time for the initial stages of the process. The first step involves negotiating agreements between all the parties concerned.

Negotiation of agreements

Most successful negotiation takes place when there is a desire to solve problems together (20). Effective problem solving involves six separate steps. Understanding these steps and knowing what to do to keep the process moving forward through these steps is the key to effective problem solving.

Step 1: Identifying the problem

A shared understanding of the nature of problems is crucial. Since health itself is a value, not a fact, different agencies are likely to have completely different views about which aspects of health are important and how health could be improved. It is vital that the different people listen to each other, and take time to understand each others' points of view. So, for example, if a public health physician goes into a meeting with the attitude that the epidemiological understanding of health gain is the only "right" way to look at health improvement, he or she will be introducing barriers straight away. Far better to describe your own position straightforwardly and accurately ("I think ...", "I believe ...") and then listen carefully and respectfully to other people's viewpoints. Structured activities could be used to explore philosophical issues related to health and health promotion and to identify the scope of the health promotion work of different agencies. These help to make it safe for people to express their views and feelings more openly. Suggestions for sources of activities are provided in the note at the end of the chapter (21).

Step 2: Generating alternative solutions

This is the creative part of problem solving. It is essential to get everyone's ideas, and to do this you must avoid, at all costs, being judgemental and critical of other people's ideas. Use techniques such as brainstorming to enable gathering a full range of alternatives. (Brainstorming is a way of gathering ideas without comment or criticism.) Clarify each others' suggestions through actively helping each other to talk and through using "active" listening skills, such as reflecting back meanings and summing up (22).

Step 3: Evaluating the alternative solutions

This is the stage when everyone must be honest in order to detect any flaws in possible solutions and any reasons why a solution might not work in practice. Assertive *I* messages alternating with "active" listening to each other are vital. It may be that a completely new solution, which proves to be the best one, is generated at this stage, or that a particular combination of solutions is the best way forward.

Step 4: Decision making

A mutual commitment to the agreed way forward is essential. If one person or agency makes the mistake of trying to push or persuade the others that their preferred solution is the best, when the others don't agree, then the whole operation will founder. People will only carry out solutions which they have freely chosen. If it is impossible to agree on a decision, return to step 1, and go through the process again.

Step 5: Implementing the solution

It is now necessary to talk about *who* does *what* by *when*? The most constructive attitude is one of complete trust that each party involved will faithfully carry out their contribution. Agree also on how you will together monitor and evaluate progress. If at any stage any party is failing to carry out his or her part of the agreement, confront with assertive *I* messages, as explained in the previous section on "How to resolve conflicts".

Step 6: Review and revise the solution

Not all solutions will turn out to be the best. It may be necessary to return for more problem solving. All the parties should understand that decisions are always open for revision, but no party can unilaterally modify a decision. Sometimes people will discover that they have over-committed themselves—or their agency—so it is important to keep the door open for revision should this happen.

Game theory

Game theory is an attempt to model the way in which humans interact with each other in a wide variety of situations, which can be applied in negotiations. One key concept of game theory is the distinction between zero sum and non-zero sum games. Zero sum games are games which assume that there are only a fixed number of possible gains which must be balanced by losses, and so when one player gains this can only be at the expense of losses by the other players (win–lose games). Non-zero sum games are those in which the total combined scores of the players can vary, thus introducing the possibility that more than one player can gain (win–win or no-lose games). Another key concept is the distinction between cooperative and non-cooperative games. Zero sum games are always non-cooperative, because for one player to win the other players have to lose. In non-zero sum games, the effect of cooperation between the players can make a radical difference to the outcomes, with cooperation enhancing the prospects of gains for all players. One of the most important implications of game theory is the recognition that although it is possible for all players to gain, these gains are seldom equal—almost always someone will make more gains than others. Accepting that this is "a fact of life" may help to make negotiating easier.

In health promotion, by working together we are seeking gains for everyone, and cooperation is essential.

An activity you could undertake: Assessing your leadership potential (23)

Answer the following quiz, by ringing the answer to each question which most closely reflects your beliefs or behaviour. This quiz is not scientific, and you should not feel discouraged by a low score. It will hopefully be a useful contribution to your self-assessment of how you need to develop your leadership potential.

1. *When new people join your organization do you*:
   (a) Wait for someone else to introduce them?
   (b) Make them feel welcome?
   (c) Find out more about them to help them fit in?
2. *Which of the following statements most closely reflects your beliefs*?
   (a) Leaders are born and not made.
   (b) Leadership is an outdated male myth.
   (c) Leaders are chosen by their followers.
3. *Confronted by difficult problems do you provide others with*:
   (a) Little help?
   (b) New ways of looking at them?
   (c) A systematic approach to problem solving?
4. *Which of the following best describes your approach to life*?
   (a) If it ain't broke don't fix it.
   (b) If you scratch my back, I'll scratch yours.
   (c) There are no failures, only learning opportunities.
5. *If you were working in a team on a difficult task would you*:
   (a) Hope someone else would tell you what to do?
   (b) Describe in glowing terms the purpose of the task?
   (c) Seek to establish deadlines and schedules?

continued on next page

continued

How to score

1. (a) 0, (b) 1, (c) 3
2. (a) 1, (b) 1, (c) 3
3. (a) 0, (b) 3, (c) 2
4. (a) 0, (b) 1, (c) 2
5. (a) 0, (b) 2, (c) 1

What your score means

Less than 2: you tend to opt out in situations requiring leadership.
2–10: you are more of a follower than a leader.
11–13: you appear to have some of the characteristics of a leader. To check this out ask some of your colleagues or staff to fill in the quiz for you.

Questions you could ask yourself

1. Identify a number of specific jobs at different levels in your organization. How well does each one meet the QWL principles for job design? Can you think of anything which could be done to improve the design of these jobs?
2. Think of one team to which you belong (as a member or a leader). What stage of team development is this team at? If it is not yet performing to its full potential, can you think of anything which could be done to help it to mature?

NOTES, REFERENCES AND FURTHER READING

(1) Reported in the *Health Service Journal* (1994) **104** (5426): 5.

(2) Higgins, J. (1994) Reformed characters. *Health Service Journal 104* (5390): 33.

(3) These characteristics are based on the findings of a survey on NHS trust leadership in Scotland, reported in:

Deffenbaugh, J. (1994) Following the leaders. *Health Service Journal* **104** (5424): 28–29

(4) Manning, K. (1994) Things to Come. *Health Service Journal* **104** (5422): 24–26.

(5) For more information on the skills of listening and helping people to talk, and on teaching and instructing, see:

Ewles, L. and Simnett, I. (3rd edn, 1995) *Promoting Health: A Practical Guide*. London: Scutari Press. Chs 8 and 11.

(6) Claxton, C.S. and Murrell, P.H. (1987) *Learning Styles: Implications for Improving Educational Practice*. ASHE-ERIC Higher Education Report No. 4. Washington, DC: Association for the Study of Higher Education.

(7) Riding, R. and Cheema, I. (1991) Cognitive styles: an overview and integration. *Educational Psychology* **11 (3 and 4)**: 193–215.

(8) For a helpful summary of those criteria which have been established for effective learning generally, see:

Miller, A. and Watts, P. (1991) *Planning and Managing Effective Professional Development for Staff Working with Children who have Special Needs*. Harlow: Longman.

For a helpful guide to study techniques, including guidance on the most effective ways of reading study materials, learning through group discussion, and writing articles, see:

Northledge, A. (1990) *The Good Study Guide*. Milton Keynes: Open University Press.

(9) Pascale argues that successful organizations develop a system that encourages constant questioning, and that leaders need to continually question their own assumptions. See:

Pascale (1991) *Managing on the Edge*. Harmondsworth: Penguin.

Ohmae has written the most practical guide to developing the higher management arts of strategic thinking. He believes that intuition and insight can be more effective in designing strategies than rational analysis, and he argues that creativity can be cultivated. The book cleverly takes apart the processes of strategic thinking, showing you how to separate the components of a problem or situation and ask the right questions. Ohmae accurately foresaw seven major changes in thinking which are influencing strategy in the 1990s. Although written in 1982 this book is still capable of changing the way you make decisions. See:

Ohmae, K. (1982) *The Mind of the Strategist: An Art of Japanese Business*. New York: McGraw Hill.

For a research-based model of effective leadership and of leadership skills, see:

Gordon, T. (1979) *Leader Effectiveness Training*. London: Futura.

(10) Gordon, T. (1979) *Leader Effectiveness Training*. London: Futura. Ch. 8.

(11) De Bono, E. (1986) *Conflicts: A Better Way to Resolve Them*. Harmondsworth: Penguin.

For open learning materials on conflict resolution, see the unit on "Negotiation", which was written by Glenn MacDonald, and is part of *Management Competencies for Health Gain* in the *Managing Health Improvement Project* (MAHIP) materials. For information about the availability of these materials, see note (8) in chapter 1.

(12) Ford, C. (1993) *A Strategy for Improving Quality of Working Life*. In Jenkins, R. and Warman, D. (eds), *Promoting Mental Health Policies in the Workplace*. London: HMSO. Ch. 8.

For further information on QWL contact Campbell Ford, ACAS, 27 Wilton Street, London, SW1 X7AZ. Telephone: 0171 210 3899.

(13) For further reading on the prevention of stress at work, see:

Warren, E. and Toll, C. (1993) *The Stress Work Book: How Individuals, Teams and Organizations Can Balance Pressure and Performance*. London: Nicholas Brealey.

(14) See, for example:

Skynner, R. and Cleese, J. (1993) *Life and How to Survive it*. London: Methuen.

(15) Belbin, R.M. (1981) *Management Teams: Why They Succeed or Fail*. Oxford: Butterworth-Heinemann.

(16) A useful game has been devised to help teams to identify these roles, and to build successful teams. See:

Platt, S. with Piepe, R. and Smyth, J. (1988) *Teams: A Game to Develop Group Skills*. Aldershot: Gower.

(17) For an introduction to team theory and to activities which will help build teams in health education and health promotion settings, see:

Rolls, E. (1992) *Team Development: A Manual of Facilitation for Health Educators and Health Promoters*. London: Health Education Authority.

For open learning materials on teamworking, see the unit on "Teambuilding" (written by Glenn MacDonald) which is part of *Management Competencies for Health Gain* in the *Managing Health Improvement Project* (MAHIP) materials. For information about the availability of these materials, see note (8) in chapter 1.

For exercises in teambuilding, see:

Maddux, R.B. (1988) *Teambuilding: An exercise in Leadership*. London: Kogan Page.

For a classic text on teambuilding, see:

Adair, J. (2nd edn, 1987) *Effective Teambuilding*. London: Pan.

For many more activities to use in teams, see:

Brandes, D. and Phillips, H. (1978) *Gamesters Handbook*. London: Hutchinson.

Brandes, D. (1983) *Gamesters Two*. London: Hutchinson.

(18) Tuckman, B.W. (1965) Developmental sequence in small groups. *Psychological Bulletin* **63**: 384–399.

See also:

Woodcock, M. (2nd edn, 1989) *Team Development Manual*. Aldershot: Gower. Ch. 3.

(19) West, M. and Anderson, N. (1994) Measures of invention: what makes one hospital management team more innovative than another? *Health Service Journal* **104** (5425): 26–27.

(20) Negotiation is the art of creating agreement on a specific issue between two (or more) parties with different views.

For a useful text on how to negotiate, see:

Hodgson, J. (1994) *Thinking on Your Feet in Negotiations: Rapid Response Tactics*. London: Pitman.

For a guide which contains all the information managers and team run a training course on negotiating, see:

Cane, S. (1994) *Ready Made Activities for Negotiating Skills*. London: Pitman.

(21) See:

Ewles, L. and Simnett, I. (3rd edn, 1995) *Promoting Health: A Practical Guide*. London: Scutari Press. Exercises in Chs 1, 2 and 3.

(22) For more information on the skills of active listening and how to help people to talk, see:

Ewles, L. and Simnett, I. (3rd edn, 1995) *Promoting Health: A Practical Guide*. London: Scutari Press. Ch. 8.

(23) This quiz is adapted from a much longer questionnaire which was compiled by James Durcan of Ashridge Management College.

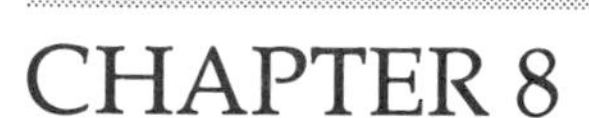

CHAPTER 8 Learning from others involved in health development

Summary

This chapter begins by looking at how a strategic approach to health promotion has developed in the UK over the 10 years from 1985 to 1995, based on the foundation of the World Health Organization's "*Health For All 2000*" movement. It moves on to consider a number of initiatives to improve health at work, and then discusses what we have learned through the development of two types of health-promoting organizations: health-promoting schools and health-promoting hospitals. A section on recommendations for the future, an activity you could undertake and some questions you could ask yourself complete the chapter.

This chapter looks at "the state of the art" in some key aspects of planning, managing, providing and evaluating health promotion. It identifies some important learning points, provides guidance and case studies, and makes some recommendations for future policy and practice. It starts by discussing the key role which the World Health Organization (WHO) has played in the evolution of health strategies and looks at how one city in England has developed and implemented a health strategy over 10 years, based on the WHO "*Health For All*" philosophy.

STRATEGIC APPROACHES TO HEALTH PROMOTION

Although we are now witnessing a much more strategic approach to health promotion, through the evolution of national and local health strategies, the WHO has been advocating such a strategic approach for some time. WHO has taken a leading role in action for health promotion since the 1970s. WHO stated in 1977, at the Thirtieth World Health Assembly, that "The main social target of governments and WHO in the coming decades should be the attainment of all citizens of the world by the year 2000 of a level of health that will permit them to lead a socially and economically productive life" (1). This was the beginning of what has come to be known as the *"Health for All"* (HFA 2000) movement which led to the development of a regional strategy for the WHO European Region in 1980 (2). This regional strategy called for fundamental changes in the health policy of member countries, including a much higher priority for health promotion and disease prevention. It called for not merely the health services but all public sectors with a potential impact on health to take positive steps to maintain and improve it. Specific regional targets were set and published in 1985 which emphasized the themes of:

- Reducing inequalities in health.
- Positive health through health promotion and disease prevention.
- Community participation.
- Cooperation between health authorities, local authorities and others with an impact on health.
- A focus on primary health care as the main basis of the health care system.

This gave impetus to the new interest in health promotion which we are now experiencing in the 1990s, with its emphasis on focusing on primary health care, health alliances, and on community participation in health promotion.

During the 1980s WHO set up the *"Healthy Cities"* movement, which focuses on action for health promotion at city level, aiming to place health high on the agenda of political decision makers, key groups in cities and the population at large (3).

The following case study briefly describes the health strategy developed by one city in England, *"Healthy Oxford 2000"*, during its first 10 years from 1985. It can be seen that the managerial approach has shifted significantly over the years to take account of political changes. The message for health managers, whether in the NHS or local government, is the same. Managers need to be clear about their goals and objectives, and use the prevailing context to continue to move towards them. Another learning point is the impetus which the new managerial climate has given to the search for more effective and efficient approaches to health promotion.

Case study: Healthy Oxford 2000 (4)

The first five years

"In 1985, a new council was elected in Oxford. It came in with the mission to challenge and change things. As far as we health managers were concerned,

continued on next page

continued

our brief was to develop and enhance the traditional environmental health services and to challenge and change the traditional approach to health provision. This entailed amongst other things:

- Breaking down the barrier that put personal health services outside local government's brief.
- Establishing a holistic approach to health.
- Opening up health decisions to the community and stimulating the community to become health activists.
- Encouraging other departments to see health 'as their business'.
- Establishing a health grants system to the voluntary sector which would not only provide cash but 'know-how' and entryism into the National Health Service.
- Democratizing health.

Generous resources in terms of extra staff and funding were given to the health managers. One of the key appointments was the establishment of a health liaison post. The council appointed a young doctor of sociology to this post. Phil was a local person whose father had been a convenor at the local car factory and therefore not surprisingly had strong connections with the trade union movement and community groups. In fact, he had for the past two years worked as coordinator of the trade unions/community 'Who Cares Campaign' set up in response to the district health authority's proposed cuts in health services. What followed was a period of intense activity, controversy and some solid achievements.

An early success was the appointment of an 'AIDS Prevention Officer' and the establishment of an AIDS Prevention Programme. This proved to be a national breakthrough in getting to grips with a hitherto 'no go' area. Over the next few years there then followed a whole range of initiatives which with the passing of time now seem a little old hat but at the time were new and exciting: health grants to voluntary organizations; the appointment of a local government nutritionist and development of healthy eating in our restaurants and pubs plus the launch of the 'non-victimizing Oxford diet'; confronting the problems of smoking at work both from the passive and the victims' points of view; an Agewell project examining the needs of carers and cared for via the doctors surgery and organizing over 50 agencies to provide support; pioneering the 'stay put' concept with the introduction of the first 'one stop shop' for the elderly house owner; 'recreation prescriptions' which brought together general practice and our recreation department; an annual health festival; a quarterly 'health tabloid' with opportunities for the public to give their views on health priorities; the establishment by the council of a bank of nurses through which we marketed and provided health screening to such companies as Marks & Spencer and Nielsons; the legitimizing of complementary medicine with the health authority. All these and others are written up in more detail elsewhere (5). Suffice it to say, that although now most of these things are no longer novel, then, as health managers in local government we were managing new and exciting phenomena.

continued on next page

continued

The style of management was 'experiential'. Put another way, in the words of the management guru Tom Peters, it was 'load, fire and aim' (6). We might not have hit the target first time but what it did was to evoke feedback which helped us to find the real target at the next attempt."

The second five years

"Things began to change from 1990. Nationally, important political changes had been taking place since 1979. For health managers in local government these were to have profound effects. The 'rate capping' which had first appeared in the Conservative manifesto in 1985 was brought into being and began to bite in 1990. This led to major cuts in resources and a close scrutiny of discretionary functions. Similarly the Audit Commission which hitherto had confined itself to fiscal propriety was tasked by government to examine management practices with a view to encouraging an approach based on the 'scientific' school of management (i.e., management by objectives). Compulsory competitive tendering, business plans, measurable performance targets and tighter management control became the managerial reference points.

So, how have these changes affected *Healthy Oxford 2000*? Paradoxically, although it has given rise to cuts and withdrawal from some areas and certainly a change in the style of management, it has acted not as a dampener but a stimulant. On the negative side we have lost some key officers and seen our local authority funding cut. However, on the positive side this has led to a search and a securing of external funding. It has also encouraged us to look for alternatives. For example, we did not have the money to establish the screening programme at a profitable level so we scrapped it and introduced with the health authority the 'Health Award' aimed at encouraging industry and commerce to an enhanced standard of health and safely plus the adopting of three personal health good practices and three environmental health good practices. This has proved remarkably successful.

Similarly, we have established with our European civic cities, plus the university, health authority, Harwell, Rover/BMW, and others, an 'Airwatch Partnership', which is proving very helpful in moving forward with tackling the problem of traffic pollution. Health 'advocacy' is now featured more strongly on our agenda. Local people have a right to health information that concerns them. In 1993 we were awarded the national award for freedom of information for work in this area.

So the changes in the managerial climate rather than dampening down *Healthy Oxford 2000* have given it new life, as can be seen in our new Health Plan. We look forward to celebrating its 10 years anniversary."

Peter Allen
October 1994

HEALTH AT WORK

> Oliver Blandford, who ran Upper Clyde Shipbuilders a couple of decades ago, had a problem with absenteeism, so he pinned up a notice, with the names of absentees, arranged under the names of their respective foremen. Naturally, some foremen had a lot more absentees than others. When they complained about being criticized, Blandford told them: "It's not criticism. I just thought you'd like to know which foremen have the fewest absentees so that you can ask them what they are doing that you're not."
>
> John Cleese (7)

WHO also recognized the critical part that workplace health promotion can play in improving the working population's health status and its role in developing an overall health-orientated culture (8). Working for improved health at work has taken high priority on the health agenda throughout the European Community and in North America and Canada in the 1990s. This is because of increased awareness of the potential effectiveness of health promotion in the workplace, not only in terms of improved employee health, but as measured by reduced sickness and absenteeism rates and improved morale and productivity (9). (The term "workplace" is used to mean the actual location where work is carried out.) However, there has been little formal evaluation (i.e, rigorously designed evaluation studies) of workplace health promotion programmes in the UK and indeed even modest in-house evaluations have been sadly lacking. There is a need to establish workplace research programmes, and to improve the ability of those responsible for health promotion in the workplace to evaluate their activities.

What we know about effective approaches to workplace health promotion comes mainly from North America, Canada, Scandinavia and Japan. Evaluation studies in these countries have shown that the best results come from comprehensive programmes that look at both the work environment, mental well-being and the reduction of stress at work, and lifestyle changes such as giving up smoking. Single-focus programmes, such as fitness testing or screening programmes, which tend to be self-selecting towards the healthier members of the workforce, have only a limited effect which is not sustained over time. The most successful programmes are those in which the workforce take an active part in deciding what programmes to introduce, and in implementing and evaluating them.

The Health Education Authority has recently undertaken a survey of workplace health promotion which provides, for the first time, a picture of what is happening in England at workplaces of all sizes and types in both the public and private sectors (10). This survey will provide a baseline measure of workplace health promotion activity in England and help the various agencies and employers working on workplace health promotion to develop more effective programmes. Key findings of the survey were:

- Overall, 40% of the workplaces surveyed (a random sample of 1344 workplaces in March and April 1992) had undertaken at least one major health-related activity in the previous year.
- A very wide range of health-related activity takes place in the workplace. Smoking, alcohol, stress, healthy eating and HIV/AIDS feature prominently.
- Larger workplaces are more likely to have more health promotion programmes, as are workplaces with recognized unions.
- In many workplaces the person responsible for health promotion has no specific training or qualification in this area.
- Consultation with the workforce before implementing health promotion activities only takes place in about half the sites.
- Those employers who had health promotional activity saw clear advantages for the organization as a whole and for employees.
- Workplaces which have no health promotion activity are small or medium sized, in the private sector, British-owned, and predominantly from distribution and catering.

Guidelines for successful workplace health promotion programmes

1. A thoroughly planned and coordinated approach is essential, with backing from senior management, and involvement of all levels of staff and managers.

   Allow plenty of time for the planning stages because it is these stages which are crucial for success. *Health At Work* programmes should be substantial and sustained over a long period of time (i.e., many years), although component projects may change with time. Programmes should be designed to meet strategic goals and objectives, in terms of both health benefits (the improved health of staff) and economic benefits (the improved performance of the business or organization concerned), which meet the expressed needs of both the employees, the employer and the corporate organization as a whole.
2. Make sure that you know what the health needs of the workforce are, and what the economic needs of the organization are, before starting a programme, then you will be able to design a programme which is

relevant to these specific needs. Examples of baseline information which you need to collect are:

- Numbers of absences due to sickness, and the reasons for these absences.
- What the priorities of the workforce are for health promotion programmes.
- Numbers of smokers.
- Numbers of employees taking regular physical exercise.
- Levels of perceived work-related stress.
- Levels of self-esteem and well-being.
- Levels of alcohol consumption.
- Ways of coping with stress.
- Accident rates.
- Perceived quality of working life.
- Perceptions on working conditions.
- Information on how work is organized, such as quality improvement management systems, team working, job design.
- Information on employee participation in policy development and work practices.
- Information on staff morale, motivation and turnover.

Collecting this information will have the added benefit of ensuring that all sectors of the workforce are involved in programme development right from the start. Regular reviews of the health needs of the workforce and the economic needs of the business will be essential as the programme unfolds.

3. Cultivate a sense of joint ownership of programmes right from the start by consulting with all those concerned (managers, occupational health staff, personnel officers, trade unions, employees, etc.) and by encouraging the active participation of all parties. Collaboration across all staff groups should be an essential and integral element of all *Health At Work* programmes. Arguably the best way to achieve this is to delegate the development, implementation and evaluation of the programme and projects to working groups or taskforces representing all sectors of the workforce. These working groups could report to a central steering group responsible for reviewing the overall strategy.
4. Be clear about the goals and objectives of health promotion programmes and ensure that there is a close fit between these and the activities you intend to undertake So, for example, if your aim is to reduce sickness absenteeism, and the main reason for absenteeism is back problems, then the focus of your health promotion programme must be on the reduction of back injuries, not on other issues. Ensure also that your programme targets and reaches those most at risk (for

example, related to the prevention of back problems, it will be important to target an NHS *Health At Work* programme at nurses).

5. Make sure that evaluation is an integral part of health promotion programmes. Decisions about what and how to evaluate must be taken at the same time as decisions to undertake a programme and what form the programme will take. Evaluate the process as well as the outcomes of your programme, and treat evaluation as an ongoing learning process, so that you review, revise and improve the programme as you go along. The sort of performance indicators which you will need to set before you start, and then monitor and review on an ongoing basis, include process and outcome measures which will answer the following questions:
   - Is the programme reaching those for whom it is intended?
   - Are people satisfied with the programme?
   - Are all the components of the programme being implemented properly?
   - Are those responsible for providing the programme competent to do so?
   - Are the resources, such as literature, used in the programme of high quality?
   - How will we know whether we are succeeding?
   - How will we know what to do next?
6. Ensure that you have high-quality programmes, through good programme management and through developing and training those who will be responsible for providing the programme.

For further information on how to manage high-quality programmes, see Chapter 4. For further information on how to evaluate programmes, including further discussion of performance indicators for *Health At Work*, see Chapter 6. For guidance on how to develop and implement workplace health policies, see the suggestion in the note at the end of the chapter (11).

Look After Your Heart workplace programme (12)

The Look After Your Heart (LAYH) programme was set up in 1987 and grew out of an earlier Look After Yourself (LAY) adult education project. It is jointly funded by the Health Education Authority and the Department of Health. It is a holistic lifestyle programme aiming to address issues as they relate to the individual person within their life context. It aims to enable people to have a better understanding of nutrition and other health topics, to take more physical activity safely, if appropriate, and to understand and handle stress. The programme includes the training of tutors from a wide variety of backgrounds. The LAYH programme is multifaceted, and one of the six building blocks is a workplace programme. A regional network of Workplace Officers take the programme into workplaces.

Health at Work in the NHS

This is an initiative launched in 1992 by the Secretary of State as part of the *Health of the Nation* strategy, and commissioned from the Health Education Authority by the NHS Executive. For the opening phase, an action pack was sent to all health authority general managers and to the chief executives of NHS Trusts, in September 1992 (13). *Health At Work in the NHS* aims to:

- Introduce a systematic healthy workplace programme throughout the NHS.
- Engage all NHS staff in health promoting activities.

This initiative builds on existing good practice and incorporates other NHS employment schemes, such as "Opportunity 2000" (14). When it was first launched, many health authorities, NHS Trusts, family health services authorities, GP practices and other NHS workplaces were already implementing policies for smoking, healthy eating and sensible drinking. A large number were also signed up to the *Look After Your Heart* workplace charter. *Health at Work in the NHS* is a long-term project building on these foundations. The aim is that the NHS becomes an "exemplar" employer, demonstrating to others that a healthy workforce benefits both individual staff members and the organization as a whole. This will help the NHS to provide better services, because healthy staff are in a better position to care for others. The *Health-Promoting Hospital* concept forms one arm of *Health at Work in the NHS* (see the section on this initiative, later in this chapter).

How healthy is the NHS workforce? The evidence suggests—not very. In 1993 the Confederation of British Industry (CBI) undertook a survey to provide evidence of the extent to which British industry is involved in promoting employees' health (15). It found that sickness absence is 41% higher in health and local authority workers than in the private sector. NHS staff lose a million working days a year from smoking-related illness alone and the cost through sickness absence is £200 million a year. Regions now have workforce health built into their contracts with the Executive, and it is beginning to roll down into service contracts, with people being nominated to take on a health at work role.

Stress at work

The National Association for Staff Support within the health care services (NASS) argues that stress at work is a cause of both physical and mental illness in NHS employees and that management style can be a cause in itself (16). The evaluation of strategies to combat workplace stress is in its infancy. Nevertheless, demands for staff support are growing and some health authorities and other employers now have well-developed systems (17). The issue has an ethical dimension in the NHS: if the NHS fails to acknowledge and take action on widely accepted determinants of organizational health, or fails to concern itself with the health of people who work in the NHS, then it is undermining its own credibility (18) One of the problems associated with many current stress management initiatives is that they focus exclusively on helping individuals to cope with stress, rather than focusing also on changing the work environment and the way work is organized. The concepts of "healthier work" and "healthier management" require promotion—working conditions and work managed and organized in such a way that they themselves contribute to good health. Interventions to help individuals cope with and manage stress are probably most effective when they are used in conjunction with organizational development and management development interventions, such as the measures to develop and manage health-promoting organizations suggested in the previous chapters of this book.

A corporate policy to reduce stress at work needs to incorporate the following (some of these have been addressed in detail in previous chapters) (19):

- An effective equal opportunities policy including fair recruitment and selection procedures.
- Good management training and development—incorporating stress management, change management, how to develop and manage health-promoting organizations, personal development and leadership development.
- Effective policies on supervision and staff appraisal/development.
- Increasing employees' control over their work and work environment, through approaches such as job design, team development, action learning sets, projects and facilitation by more experienced and able staff or managers.
- Life skills training for the workforce (this is discussed further in Chapter 9).
- Systems that assess the impact on health of the whole organization, as well as of its individual units, and identify ways to improve health through "healthier work" and "healthier management".
- Policies for sickness absence, including monitoring of records.
- Substance abuse policies.

- Information on and access to confidential counselling and support groups.

For a discussion on the ACAS "Quality of Working Life" initiative, which aims to prevent and reduce stress at work through, for example, applying principles of good job design, see Chapter 7. MIND has produced an excellent information pack for employers, which sets out a model code of good practice in recruitment and selection aiming to reduce discrimination against people with mental health problems (20). It includes a useful model equal opportunities policy statement, which is set out in the following box.

A model equal opportunities policy statement

"______ is an equal opportunity employer and will apply objective criteria to assess merit. It aims to ensure that no job or applicant or employee receives less favourable treatment on the grounds of race, colour, nationality, religion, ethnic or national origin, sex, marital status, sexual orientation, physical or mental disability or is disadvantaged by conditions or requirements which cannot be shown to be justifiable.

Selection criteria and procedures will be reviewed frequently to ensure that individuals are selected, promoted and treated on the basis of their relevant merits and abilities. All employees will be given equal opportunity and, where appropriate and possible, special training, facilities and support to enable them to progress both within and outside the organization. ______ is committed to a programme of action to make this policy fully effective."

For further reading on mental health in the workplace, and for training materials which can be used both for self-directed learning and for training supervisors and managers in stress management, see the note at the end of the chapter (21).

DEVELOPING HEALTH-PROMOTING SCHOOLS

The importance of the whole school in providing a health-promoting environment through a "health-promoting school" was first highlighted in the UK by a Scottish Health Education Group report (22). The Health Education Authority is now participating in a European Network of Health-Promoting Schools Project together with the Department for Education and in liaison with the National Curriculum Council. The Advisory Council on Alcohol and Drug Education (TACADE) has also supported schools (23).

Some local education authorities and health authorities have launched a "*healthy schools award*" which recognizes the achievements of a school in making school life a health-promoting experience for all children and adults who teach, learn and work in it. So, for example, Hampshire County Council and Wessex Institute of Public Health Medicine have jointly developed a *healthy schools award* through the work of an alliance of pilot schools representing key stages 1–4, and health professionals, education inspectors and advisers (24). Schools receiving the award must demonstrate progress on performance indicators related to nine key statements (key results areas). These are:

1. The school should be working towards the National Curriculum Guidance Document No. 5 (Health Education). Its policies and programmes should be coordinated, comprehensive and progressive, and be reflected in the School Development Plan.
2. Policies should reflect the school as part of the community.
3. The school should be working towards a smoke-free environment.
4. Pupils should be educated and encouraged to make healthy food choices.
5. The school should offer a wide range of physical activities which are accessible to all and in which working towards health becomes an important cultural practice within the school (National Curriculum Physical Education Statutory Orders).
6. Schools should encourage young people to take responsibility for their own health.
7. The school should be a health-promoting workplace for staff.
8. The school should promote a generally stimulating, clean, safe and tidy environment.
9. There should be equal opportunity and access to health education for all who teach, learn, and work in the school.

The following case study illustrates the work of one school in these nine key areas.

Developing a health-promoting school: Dorcan School, Swindon, Wiltshire (25)

Dorcan School is an 11–16 comprehensive school maintained by the Education Committee of Wiltshire County Council. It opened in 1970 and was designed as a purpose-built community comprehensive school for the urban villages of Eldene, Liden, Covingham and Nythe. The joint provision with the Borough of Thamesdown provides swimming pool, squash courts, floodlit artificial pitch,

continued on next page

continued

tennis courts, gymnasium, sports hall, all-weather cricket pitch and "redgra" athletics surfaces. These are in addition to the usual range of soccer and rugby pitches and general play areas. All these facilities are available to Dorcan students during the day and are extensively used in the evening by the general public. The site is run by three agencies: the school itself, Wiltshire Youth and Community Service and Thamesdown Borough Council.

Dorcan was one of the pilot schools involved in developing the "*healthy schools award*". The initiatives it has taken to contribute to the nine key areas include:

1. "*Its policies and programmes should be coordinated, comprehensive and progressive ...*"

   A comprehensive system for coordination has been developed which is pupil-centred and radiates out from the pupil through the tutor system (which forms part of the Faculty of Personal Development and Support) to all key activity areas, including:
   - National Curriculum subjects.
   - Curriculum changes, with the introduction of General National Vocational Qualifications (GNVQ), are under consideration.
   - Curriculum continuity (including integration of health education across the curriculum).
   - Primary/tertiary transfer.
   - Careers, including school-based provisions and links with the Careers Service.
   - Pastoral care, including links with educational welfare officers, child and family guidance, police, social services counsellor, educational psychologist, and school-based provisions for those with special educational needs.
   - Extracurricular activities, including sport, drama, music, art club, conservation group and public speaking.

   All areas of the school activities contribute to health education, with particular emphasis coming from physical education, science, food technology and the pastoral system. The entire curriculum has been mapped to integrate and coordinate these experiences. A cross-curriculum group has representatives from each faculty in the school and focuses on issues such as careers, the school environment and health. Each year a different theme is highlighted for particular emphasis, whilst ensuring that the previous years' themes are sustained.

2. "*Policies should reflect the school as part of the wider community.*"

   Thamesdown Borough Council has an "active lifestyles" programme and the approach to physical education in the school mirrors this. Links have been established with the health promotion programmes of Swindon Health Promotion Department. A visit to the Thamesdown Borough "Health Hydro" (which offers a range of healthy activities including access to alternative medicine) was organized for all staff who work on the site, including teaching staff, cleaners, caterers and youth and community workers.

continued on next page

continued

Vandalism on the site has decreased and this may be related to liaison with the community policeman who lives and works in the area and frequently visits the school, and to environmental activities which have highlighted the responsibility of pupils to look after the school environment (see point 8).

Links have been established with local businesses and industry. So, for example, Rover apprentices designed the school lecture theatre for a change of use. Neighbourhood engineers from the Post Office Research Centre have worked with pupils in the classroom.

Good links have been forged with partner primary schools. A "primary classroom" in the Dorcan School enables primary school pupils to study at the school for a day, and to work with Dorcan staff, prior to transfer. New pupils have a full induction programme.

The school's involvement in community projects has been recognized through the Civic Trust Award.

3. "*The school should be working towards a smoke free environment.*"

   The whole site is a no-smoking area, although two areas have been set aside as designated smoking areas. One of these is off the staff room, but since the introduction of the smoking policy use of this has declined and no members of staff regularly use this now. The other area is used by the general public who have access to site facilities.

4. "*Pupils should be educated and encouraged to make healthy food choices.*"

   In food technology, healthy food is stressed and all pupils, whether boys or girls, plan, prepare, cook and eat meals. "Non-chip" days and "Italian weeks" have featured in the menus provided by contract caterers. However, contract caterers can only sell what is profitable, and teachers would prefer a set menu, with options, but offering a balanced meal. This is seen as particularly important for those pupils receiving free school meals, and the head teacher is exploring ways of enhancing provision in consultation with the catering company.

5. "*The school should offer a wide range of physical activities.*"

   Besides offering a wide range of sporting and physical activities at school, including incorporating swimming in the year 7 programme, the school has undertaken a number of specific initiatives to encourage pupil awareness of, and access to, a wide range of physical activities. So, for example, the school "sports day" has been developed into a "sport and health day". In the morning pupils have the opportunity to participate in activities such as sailing and ice-skating, and in the afternoon the athletics championships are held. All pupils participate in "health-related fitness" courses during Key Stages 3 and 4. This involves planning a "menu", designing their own fitness programme and keeping a diary of fitness activities. Pupils have been offered opportunities to learn relaxation and massage techniques and visit fitness centres off the school site.

continued on next page

continued

However, due to National Curriculum time demands a timetabled programme entitled "Lifestyles", in which pupils covered such areas as first aid, life saving and community work, has had to be dropped from the school's curriculum.

6. "*Schools should encourage young people to take responsibility for their own health.*"

   This is reinforced during the tutorial programme, when issues such as positive health, self-esteem, social well-being and personal responsibility are opened up. Pupils are responsible for maintaining the environment of their own tutor group space. Health promotion literature is available to pupils. A student ethos policy is being developed and all pupils complete a Personal Development Plan (PDP) which contributes to the National Record of Achievement (NRA).

7. "*The school should be a health-promoting workplace for staff.*"

   Health classes have been run for staff, including bereavement classes, relaxation classes and well-women classes. Opportunities to learn relaxation and massage techniques are being offered to staff, to help them to cope with stress.

8. "*The school should promote a generally stimulating, clean, safe and tidy environment.*"

   Pupils are actively involved in the design and management of the school environment. Paper and cans are recycled (with several banks for cans on site). The concept of "graffiti" has been used positively by pupils to produce graffiti boards which improve the school environment. A wildlife conservation area has been designed and developed by the pupils, with the help of a JCB digger loaned by a parent. An anti-bullying code is actively promoted and states that: "As members of the Dorcan School community, we all have a responsibility to create a safe environment where we can work, study and play without fear." The school's environmental education programme has been recognized through the Royal Anniversary Trust's Schools Award.

9. "*There should be equal opportunity and access to health education for all who teach, learn and work in the school.*"

   The school's equal opportunities policy is expressed in a variety of ways. So, for example, girls play football and rugby and boys play hockey. At Key Stage 4, girls can opt for basketball and cricket. All pupils taking food technology plan, prepare, cook and eat meals. The school's achievements in equalizing opportunities have been recognized through the national Menerva Education Trust Award 1994.

For further reading on school health education, see the suggestions in the note at the end of the chapter (26).

DEVELOPING HEALTH-PROMOTING HOSPITALS

The conceptual framework for health-promoting hospitals evolved from the WHO *Health For All* strategy together with the directives set out in the *Ottawa Charter for Health Promotion* and the *Budapest Declaration* (27). A European Network of Health-Promoting Hospitals was established by WHO in 1991 (28). In England, the Preston Acute Hospitals Trust (Sharoe Green Hospital and the Royal Preston Hospital) are the official WHO pilot scheme. The progress they have made so far is summarized in the following box.

Building health-promoting hospitals in Preston (29)

The development of health-promoting hospitals in Preston has been based on a clear management philosophy:

1. The success of the strategy will be conditional upon the organization encouraging freedom of thinking at all levels among the staff.
2. The organization needs to know where it is going to create successful organizational change.
3. The active participation of staff and a management philosophy which encourages this are essential for success.
4. The promotion of health must become part of he way the public perceives the hospital.

The hospitals have adopted five health-promotion projects:

1. *A "healthy environment" in a health-promoting hospital*: this project is examining and improving the facilities available to staff. Evaluation and monitoring have been built in at the start of various initiatives promoted by *Health At Work in the NHS*. The occupational health department has bought screening equipment and "Wellscreen" computer software to monitor and record staff health, and a baseline study of 10% of staff at the two hospitals has begun. Exercise is being encouraged by the purchase of free and reduced price admissions to local leisure centres and a cycle loan scheme (with helmets) for employees to travel the mile between the two hospital sites.
2. *A review of the storage, collection, transport and disposal of clinical waste*: this project aims to improve the environmental impact of the hospitals. A baseline study is establishing "where we are now" and an intervention study will use the results to produce measurable improvements. Current steps include the introduction of new lockable containers which minimize manual handling of waste, thus reducing the risk of accidents. An environmental liaison officer has been appointed to implement the intervention study and to assist in research, training and audit.

continued on next page

continued

3. *The management of post-coronary patients*: one objective of this project is to assess the impact on hospital staff attitudes as post-coronary care is extended, and as patient and carer are exposed to increased understanding of the illness through educational programmes. Ex-members of the rehabilitation programmes are involved with a schools roadshow, and thus a long-term cycle is completed by giving children the means of preventing themselves from becoming occupants of the coronary care unit.
4. *Prevention of accidents through self-care*: Preston has an innovative accident and emergency department which was one of the sites earmarked by the Department of Health in 1991 as exhibiting good practice. The department aims to develop an information service and a data bank on the occurrence of accidents in the area, and use this work with the County Council to prevent accidents in the future.
5. *The health-promoting hospital in the community*: this project is exploring the practical possibility of using a health-promoting hospital as a point of entry into the community for the purpose of creating a network of "health-promoting organizations".

The newest setting (30) to be taken up by WHO, as a way of making health the focus of organizational development, is the prison (31). Five health-promoting prisons have been chosen by the prison service in England and Wales: Wayland near Thetford in Norfolk, Woodhill in Milton Keynes, Lindholme near Doncaster, Styal women's prison in Cheshire and Thorncross young offenders' institution near Warrington. Health promotion is part of the corporate plan for each of these prisons and has been written into the governors' contracts as a top priority. This is hitherto uncharted territory, and it remains to be seen how far the principles of equity and empowerment central to the *Health for All* philosophy can be adopted by prisons.

RECOMMENDATIONS FOR THE FUTURE

Developing health-promoting workplaces should be part of a wider movement to develop health-promoting organizations and businesses. Workplaces cannot be healthy unless they are part of "healthy firms" or "healthy institutions". Developing healthy firms needs a "pincer movement" with "top down" health strategies and a changed management style and corporate climate, based on a horizontal rather than a vertical organizational structure. Full participation by all employees will produce "bottom-up" ideas through activities such as projects, action learning sets and the implementation of quality improvements by the workforce. Working towards healthy organizations should be based on a positive vision of what such organizations will be like, and what the experience of working in them will feel like. The more we get clear about our vision of healthy organizations, for all who work in them and for all those associated with them, as suppliers, purchasers, customers, patients, clients or students, the more we shall understand what are the steps necessary to create them. This positive approach should replace the current "problem"-orientated approach of much health at work activity, which focuses just on how to reduce problems such as stress, sickness absences and accidents, rather than on positive health. However, the new approach should not make the mistake of focusing just on how *individuals* can adopt healthy lifestyles (a weakness of the Look After Your Heart programme). Rather, the focus should be on improving work in a number of key results areas, such as the following.

Key results areas for the work of health-promoting organizations

- The organization should play an active role in developing and contributing to the wider community of which it is a part.
- The organization should have effective policies on equal opportunities, supervision, staff appraisal and staff development and training, which include a focus on the implications of these policies for health development.
- Staff at all levels should have access to education and training related to health development, including personal development (such as life skills training) and, when appropriate, professional development, leadership development and management development.
- The organization should have a range of health policies, such as policies on smoking, physical activity, substance abuse, lifting, health and safety, healthy eating and HIV/AIDS.
- There should be equal opportunity and access to a range of health promotion programmes for all who study, visit, use or work in the organization.
- All health promotion programmes should be of high quality, through focusing on management quality, professional quality, and quality of participation by the workforce and customers (or clients/patients or students).
- All workplaces should be health-promoting, through the adoption of "healthy" management practices and through "healthy" organizational structures and processes.

- All workplaces should be stimulating, as clean as practicable, safe and tidy.
- Steps should be taken to design, manage and conserve the workplace environment so that it is healthy and sustainable.

Each organization will need to identify appropriate performance indicators to measure progress in these nine key results areas. Awards for "healthy firms" and "healthy organizations" could be offered by health alliances between local chambers of commerce, local training and enterprise councils, local employers, local schools and colleges, local authorities and health authorities/health commissions. With the move to care in the community, the development of health-promoting residential homes for the elderly, for children in care and for those with learning disabilities and mental health problems should be one of the key targets for the work of such health alliances. Another key target should be to help small businesses to become health-promoting. Small businesses will require help with training for health promoters. Identification and sharing of resources may be one possibility. A third key target must be the development of health-promoting GP practices and primary health care.

The work ongoing in moving towards health-promoting schools and health-promoting hospitals means that we increasingly have access to models which can be applied to other types of businesses and settings. The success of this approach to health development depends crucially on the success of our efforts to empower people, whether they are patients, clients, students or employees. In the past, treatment and care and management practices have been "disempowering"—resulting in a burgeoning welfare state and dependence on professionals. Using effective ways to share power with people for better health lies at the heart of health promotion and is the subject of the final chapter.

An activity you could undertake: Measuring and making progress towards a health-promoting organization

(a) Identify pilot performance indicators for each of the nine key results areas for health-promoting organizations, suggested in this chapter, which are relevant to the work of your organization. The following example provides some suggestions for performance indicators related to one of the key results areas:

Key results area: all workplaces should be health-promoting, through the adoption of healthy management practices and through healthy organizational structures and processes.

continued on next page

continued

In what ways does the organization ensure that:

1. It has a management philosophy which is clear about the overall purpose of the organization, promotes a widely shared vision of a healthier future, and a set of values and principles which govern the way it operates?
2. All those who work in, use, or are associated with the organization are active participants in the evolution of health policies and programmes, right from the start?
3. It has an "organic" structure based on the work of semi-autonomous teams?
4. Teams are developed so that they are highly competent at health promotion work, including evaluation and quality improvement?
5. Effective communication takes place so that work is coordinated, people know what is going on and what is expected of them, morale is high because everyone is working together for a healthier future, and active participation by staff means that ideas for improving practice quickly spread throughout the organization?
6. A research-based approach is used, so that health promotion work is based on the best "state of the art"?

(b) Use your pilot performance indicators in workshops with staff (it may need more than one workshop). Ask the staff to choose one key results area which interests them, and to divide into groups, one group working on each key results area. Each group should then:

1. Rate the performance of your organization on each of the performance indicators related to their chosen key results area (with 0 representing extremely poor performance, and 10 representing excellent performance). Each group should try to reach a consensus on their rating for each performance indicator, but should also record and report on any disagreements.
2. Suggest how the performance indicators could be improved.
3. Suggest what might be the steps to improve performance in this key results area.

(c) Share the findings of each group in a plenary session. Then develop an action plan through identifying:

- The views of staff on the top priorities for action.
- Any areas over which the workers have control and could take action on right away.
- Areas which require support or approval from top management and how that will be sought and pursued.

Questions you could ask yourself

1. How do you think that the workplace health promotion programmes of your organization could be improved?
2. What could you do to ensure that any of these improvements are implemented?

NOTES, REFERENCES AND FURTHER READING

(1) WHO resolution WHO 30.43, quoted in:

WHO Regional Office for Europe (1985) *Targets for Health For All*. Copenhagen: WHO. p. 1.

(2) WHO Regional Office for Europe (1985) *Targets for Health For All*. Copenhagen: WHO.

There is a UK network for all those who are committed to pursuing the WHO HFA 2000 strategy. For further information on this network, contact UK Health for All Network, PO Box 101, Liverpool, L69 5BE. Telephone: 0151 231 1009.

(3) Kickbush, I. (1989) Healthy cities: a working project and a growing movement. *Health Promotion* **4** (2): 77.

Ashton, J. and Seymour, H. (1988) *The New Public Health*. Milton Keynes: Open University Press. Ch. 9.

(4) This case study was written by Peter Allen, Deputy City Environmental Health Officer for Oxford City, and is reproduced with kind permission from Oxford City Council. For further information contact: Environmental Health Department, Thomas Hull House, 1 Bonn Square, Oxford OX1 1QH. Telephone: 01865 249811.

(5) Allen, P. (1992) *Off the Rocking Horse*. London: Greenprint.

(6) Peters, T. (1989) *Thriving on Chaos*. London: Pan Books in association with Macmillan.

(7) Skynner, R. and Cleese, J. (1993) *Life and How to Survive It*. London: Methuen. p. 127.

(8) World Health Organization (1988) *Health Promotion for Working Populations*. Report of a WHO Expert Committee: Technical Report Series NO. 765. Geneva: World Health Organization.

WHO have published the results of a survey of health promotion in European organizations:

Malzon, R.A. and Lindsay, G.B. (1992) *Health Promotion at the Worksite: A Brief Survey of Large Organizations in Europe*. Copenhagen: European Occupational Health Series No. 4.

(9) The benefits of health promotion at work are well established in the USA and Canada, and reviews of the literature identify the major benefits as a significant decrease in absenteeism and staff turnover, and significant increases in productivity and morale. See, for example:

Bertera, R.I. (1990) The effects of workplace health promotion on absenteeism and employment costs in a large industrial population. *American Journal of Public Health* **80** (9): 307–327.

For an extremely useful and comprehensive review of the literature on workplace health promotion, with a particular focus on smoking and stress, see:

Directorate of Health Policy and Public Health (1993) *Workplace Health Promotion: A Review of the Literature.* Oxford: Oxford Regional Health Authority.

Copies of this review can be obtained from Health of the Nation Regional Unit, Oxford Regional Health Authority, Old Road, Headington, Oxford OX3 7FL. Telephone: 01865 742277.

This review suggests that there is some evidence from the literature that health promotion programmes, may not be reaching all sectors of the workforce, and that an inverse care law may be operating, with those in least need of health promotion being the most likely to use facilities and programmes. The authors suggest that rather than offering general programmes targeted at the whole workforce, it may be of more value to target high-risk groups.

Of the research studies that have looked at the economic benefits to be derived from health promotion programmes, most have shown them to have reduced staff turnover, reduced absenteeism, improved productivity, reduced frequency of accidents/injuries, reduced recruitment costs and improved corporate image. For a brief review of the literature on workplace health promotion, see:

Department of Health (1994) *The Health of the Nation Workplace Task Force Report.* London: Department of Health.

Copies of this report can be obtained from: Department of Health, Wellington House, 133–155 Waterloo Road, London SE1 8UG. Telephone: 0171 972 2000.

(10) Health Education Authority (1993) *Health Promotion in the Workplace: A Summary.* London: Health Education Authority.

(11) Ewles, L. and Simnett, I. (3rd edn, 1995) *Promoting Health: A Practical Guide.* London: Scutari Press. Ch. 13.

(12) Further information can be obtained from the HEA Business Unit at Christ Church College, Canterbury, Kent, CT1 1QU. Telephone: 01227 455564. The HEA Business Unit supports the work of health educators in the workplace. Through a network of over 200 trained tutors, it provides employers with a range of health promotion services throughout England, including workshops and training for staff responsible for in-house health promotion activities. It also produces a regular *Health at Work* newsletter.

(13) Health Education Authority (1992) *Health at Work in the NHS Action Pack.* London: Health Education Authority.

This has been followed by a computerized resource pack:

Health Education Authority (1994) *Working Well: A Guide to Success.* London: Health Education Authority.

(14) Opportunity 2000 is the government-backed campaign for a more woman-friendly workforce, launched by John Major in 1991. Member companies have on average 25% women at managerial level, compared with 9.5% in UK top companies as a whole. However, take-up rates for new flexible practices such as extended maternity and paternity leave, job sharing and more flexible hours remain disappointingly low. Many would argue that only with tax relief on child care and more state-funded nursery school places will Opportunity 2000 begin to make a real impact on the performance of female workers.

(15) This survey has not yet been published in its final form, but its findings are discussed in:

Department of Health (1994) *The Health of the Nation: Workplace Task Force Report*. London: Department of Health.

This document is available from Department of Health, Health Promotion (Administrative) Division, Wellington House, 133–155 Waterloo Road, London SE1 8UG. Telephone: 0171 972 2000.

(16) See:

National Association for Staff Support (1992) *The Costs of Stress and the Costs and Benefits of Stress Management*. Woking: NASS.

Copies of this briefing document can be obtained from General Secretary, National Association for Staff Support, 9 Caradon Close, Woking, Surrey GU21 3DU.

(17) See, for example:

Millar, B. (1994) Listen very carefully: staff support schemes can save lives and money, but they are far from universal in the NHS. *Health Service Journal* **104** (5386): Special Report on Human Resources, 10–11.

(18) George, J. (1990) Why stress is a management issue. *Health Manpower Management* December: 17–19.

(19) O'Leary, L. (1993) Mental health at work. *Occupational Health Review* September/October: 24–26.

(20) MIND (1991) *Action Pack on Mental Health and Employment: A Guide to Good Practice*. London: MIND.

For further information contact MIND (National Association for Mental Health), 22 Harley Street, London W1N 2ED.

(21) The Department of Health's Mental Health Interagency Group (which includes representatives of the Department of Employment, the CBI, the Institute of Personnel and Development, Health and Safety Executive, Health Education Authority, TUC, ACAS and the Federation of Small Businesses) has produced a guide for small to medium-sized businesses:

Department of Health (1994) *The ABC Guide to Mental Health in the Workplace*. London: Department of Health.

For further information on the guide, write to Dr Elaine Gadd, Department of Health, Room 307, Wellington House, 133–155 Waterloo Road, London SE1 8UG.

For a review of the literature on interventions to control stress at work, see:

Directorate of Health Policy (1994) *Workplace Health Promotion: A Review of the Literature*. Oxford: Oxford Regional Health Authority.

For information about how to obtain this review document, see note (9).

For training and self-directed learning material, see:

Sills, M. and Aris, A. (1994) *Positive Stress at Work*. London: Health Education Authority.

(22) Young, I. and Williams, T. (1989) *The Healthy School*. Edinburgh: Scottish Health Education Group.

Scottish Health Education Group/Scottish Consultative Council on the Curriculum (1990) *Promoting Good Health*: Proposals for Action in Schools. Edinburgh: SHEG.

(23) See:

TACADE (1993) *Health Promoting Schools: A DIY Training Manual for Staff INSET*. Salford: TACADE.

For information about the availability of this manual, contact TACADE, 1 Hulme Place, The Crescent, Salford M5 4QA. Telephone: 0161 745 8925.

TACADE is a national organization, established in 1968. It is a charity, working in the field of health, personal and social education to produce resource materials and training courses. It also works on a consultancy basis with a wide range of statutory and voluntary agencies and supports a variety of research projects in alcohol and drug education.

(24) See the booklet:

Wessex Institute of Public Health Medicine and Hampshire County Council Education Department (1993) *Healthy Schools Award*.

(25) This case study is based on interviews with Dorcan School staff and is reproduced by kind permission of the Dorcan School.

(26) Davies, G. and Williams, E. (1994) *Health Education for Key Stages 3 and 4: A Handbook for Teachers*. Hemel Hempstead: Simon & Schuster.

National Curriculum Council (1990) *Curriculum Guidance 5: Health Education*. York: National Curriculum Council.

Available from National Curriculum Council, 15–17 New Street, York YO1 2RA.

For training materials intended to help teachers and health service staff to work together to promote the health of children, see:

Williams, T. Wetton, N. and Moon, A. (1990) *Promoting our Children's Health in Schools: A Working Partnership*. London: Health Education Authority.

See also the section on "Developing life skills" in Chapter 9.

(27) The first International Conference on Health Promotion took place in Ottawa on the 21 November 1986 and presented a charter for action to achieve *Health For All* by the year 2000 and beyond. It stated that:

> The fundamental conditions and resources for health are peace, shelter, education, food, income, a stable ecosystem, sustainable resources, social justice and equity. Improvement in health requires a secure foundation in these basic prerequisites.

Health promotion action is seen as involving activity on a number of fronts, including healthy public policy, taking care of each other, our communities and our natural environment, strengthening community action and learning opportunities for health, developing personal and social skills, and moving the role of the health sector increasingly in a health promotion direction, beyond its responsibility for providing clinical and curative services.

In June 1991 WHO held a business meeting on healthy hospitals, which resulted in the *Budapest Declaration on Health-promoting Hospitals.* Hospitals participating in the WHO health-promoting hospital network must meet the following criteria:

1. Consistency with contemporary health and ecological messages, such as smoke-free zones, healthy eating and healthy working conditions.
2. Client satisfaction—meeting the needs and wishes of patients and their families.
3. Create supportive, humane and stimulating lively environments for all patients, staff and visitors.
4. Use the hospital's potential to develop skills for life, rehabilitation and positive health practices.
5. Strive to make the health promoting hospital a model for healthy services and workplaces.
6. Improve the participation of patients and staff in the management of the hospital.
7. Review and improve all rules, codes, organizational systems and methods of communication so that they contribute to the improved health of patients, staff and patients' families and carers.

(28) For a report on the WHO network, see:

Harrison, D. and Ashcroft, S. (1994) Health-promoting hospitals: early warning systems. *Health Service Journal* **104** (5422): 28–30.

(29) The information in this case study is based on the report of an HEA-funded conference held in Preston, April 1993:

Health Education Authority (1993) *Health Promoting Hospitals: Principles and Practice.* London: HEA.

In addition it draws on the newsletter of the *Preston Health Promoting Hospitals*, No. 1, Summer 1994. This newsletter is available from HPH Information Line, Preston Health Promotion Unit, Sharoe Green Hospital, Watling Street Road, Fulwood, Preston PR2 4DX. Telephone: 01772 711223.

See also:

NHS Executive (1994) *The Health of the Nation: Health Promoting Hospitals.* London: Department of Health.

(30) The word "setting" is used for places where people work, rest and play. WHO has pioneered a "settings" approach which looks at population groups in their natural setting, for example the family, school, hospital, workplace or prison, and identifies their needs for better health in each setting.

(31) These developments were reported at an international conference on "healthy settings" at the University of Central Lancashire in November 1993. A full report of the conference is available from Denise Richardson at the University of Central Lancashire, Preston. Telephone: 01772 893406.

CHAPTER 9 Involving local people in health development

Summary

This chapter starts by looking at the skills and attitudes required to genuinely empower local people to take charge of their own, and their family's and community's, health and well-being. It continues by suggesting two approaches that health promoters could adopt in order to change their relationship with clients and be more effective: first through understanding themselves and their clients better, and second by developing the skills required to use new behavioural techniques such as solution-focused therapy. It then discusses the pivotal role of the GP as the gateway to health promotion and the key part the extended primary health care team has to play in providing a wide range of health promotion activities at neighbourhood level. It moves on to discuss how we can extend our outreach with health promotion, so that individuals, groups and communities become active participants. It ends with some concluding thoughts from the author and an activity you could undertake.

Getting people involved in health development means changing their behaviour, from being passive to actively participating in efforts to improve their own, and others', health. Health professionals may tend to assume that everyone *wants* better health, because health is something that they value. This is far from the truth. There are, in reality, many powerful forces which encourage people to be sick, and reward people for being unhealthy. The key to getting people to work for better health lies in improving their motivation to do so. This means that health promoters must have the skills to do this, and must make this a key component of their practice, along with the technical or professional functions of their particular occupation.

In this chapter I explore what these skills are and how health promoters can use them to best effect. I point out that these skills are essentially the same ones as those required by people to promote their own, and their family's, health: life skills in how to relate to each other in a mutually beneficial way. So, if health promotion practitioners can change their behaviour and relate to their clients through using these new behavioural techniques, they will be encouraging an uplifting cycle, through which their clients gain confidence in themselves and learn the life skills needed to run their lives more effectively. The same life skills are also used in the effective management and leadership of health development, and I focused on the use of some of these in those contexts, in Chapters 3, 4 and 7.

Through our socialization, we have all learned some ineffective ways of relating to, and communicating with, each other (1). By adopting new approaches we shall all benefit, and some of the "cankers" institutionalized in our society, such as racism and sexism, will begin to break down. We need "new leadership", "new management" and, in addition, "new health promotion practice" and "new life skills", all working together to break down these barriers to better health (2).

Thus, for example, Lord Woolf emphasizes the importance of tackling one of the causes of the breakdown in social behaviour which is concerning governments worldwide—the total, or partial, failure of relationships between individuals, communities and institutions—in proposals for a radical new approach to the criminal justice system (3). The emphasis in this new approach is on preventing crime, resolving conflicts, promoting relationships based on dignity and respect for all human beings, and using "cautioning plus" penalties whenever possible—penalties under which a caution is coupled with an undertaking by the offender to do something to repair the damage to the victim. Reform of court proceedings for young offenders to make them less confrontational and more of a "conference" is also needed.

According to Christopher Brown, the director of the National Society for the Prevention of Cruelty to children (NSPCC), which is launching a three-year campaign to change attitudes towards children: "We need to change the culture of harmful behaviour within the family and prevent it becoming a tradition that is passed on down through generations" (4). A poll conducted for the NSPCC showed that 27% of 1032 adults questioned remembered being constantly or frequently criticized by their fathers and 23% by their mothers. Thirty-five per cent were never or rarely hugged or kissed by their fathers, and 18% said their mothers showed a similar lack of affection.

EMPOWERING PEOPLE FOR BETTER HEALTH

The goal of health promotion is to raise the level of wellness in individuals, families and communities. The means to this goal is through enabling people to take increased responsibility for, and to have more control over, their own and their family's and community's health and well-being. The whole way the health and caring professions have been trained, and have perceived their role, in the past, has militated against this (5). People have been cared *for*, not *about*. Goals and objectives, care and health promotion plans, have all been set by the professionals, *not* by the people concerned. What the people concerned do get is plenty of interest shown in them and their condition or problems, lots of attention, and lots of things done *for* them or *to* them. So, the professionals are active and in control; the public are passive, dependent and even, sometimes, grateful. Many people will not be dissatisfied with these arrangements, as long as the benefits (attention, care, concern, income support, health and welfare provisions, etc.) continue to roll in, and therefore will have little incentive to change. Indeed the costs of change could be perceived as very high: taking responsibility can be a frightening prospect, particularly for people whose self-esteem and self-confidence have been eroded. If we are not to fall into the trap of "blaming the victim" for their plight, what can we do instead to reverse this situation?

One thing we can do is to change the way we relate to our clients, patients, employees, customers and students. Using the change equation (see the section in Chapter 2 on "Key factors for successful development"), we need to:

- Increase people's dissatisfaction with things as they are now.
- Increase people's vision of what a healthier future will be like and the benefits it will bring.
- Ensure that people have the ability to take a small, acceptable first step.
- Reduce the perceived costs of change.

At the same time we need to stop behaving in harmful ways:

- Stop telling people what *we* (the professionals) think they should do ("stop smoking", "take more exercise", "take it easy", etc.).
- Stop trying to persuade people to do what *we* think they should do, when they are not ready to change.
- Stop trying to involve them in *our* plans for their development.

Telling people what to do and persuading people to do what we have decided is best for them, when they don't agree, are both intrinsically interventions which lessen the power people have over their own lives (they are "disempowering"). Fortunately, we now have at our disposal skills and techniques which are intrinsically empowering, for all the parties concerned, and it is to these we must turn to "operationalize" the change equation. These new concepts and methods lie at the heart of improving the quality and effectiveness of face-to-face health promotion. Using them may initially be very difficult and uncomfortable for the health promoter, because they involve respecting the autonomy of the client (while this is not always possible, for example it may not be possible, or ethical, when someone has a life-threatening condition such as anorexia, it often is not done even when it is possible). It means sometimes accepting that clients may choose to continue to behave in ways which are considered to be "unhealthy" by the health promoter. It is hard for health promoters to accept the validity of such outcomes which may cut across the norms and values of the disciplines in which they have been trained. For a detailed discussion on education, autonomy and empowerment, see the suggestion in the note at the end of the chapter (6).

Health promotion is not an add-on extra to treatment or care. It is an integral part of the process. I shall illustrate this with reference to treatment.

- First, part of treatment is to explain what will be done, what it will feel like, and what will be the consequences (this is *health education* through providing *health information*).
- Second, treatment also may require education of patients so that they can take responsibility for, and manage, their own condition (in patients with chronic conditions such as diabetes and asthma). The health education necessary to achieve this goes beyond information giving, so that patients learn the *health skills* to manage their condition.
- Third, treatment involves educating patients about how to ensure that their problem is prevented in future, through encouraging them to change their risk behaviours (such as learning how to lift properly, adopt the correct posture, and take healthy exercise, in patients with back problems). (Tudor Hart refers to this as *"anticipatory care"*, because it is anticipating patients' needs to build a healthier future (7)). The third component of health education is vital because it helps people not to become dependent on professionals (returning again and again with conditions linked to risk behaviours) and to learn how to take responsibility for promoting their own health. So, part of treatment is about helping and encouraging behaviour change, through increasing self-control—the control patients have over their own behaviour. It is orientated round building a healthier future, rather than focusing on current problems. It involves helping people to develop *life skills* (such as how to be assertive, how to make choices and decisions, how to communicate well and how to relate to others) as well as *health skills*.

Health and social care practitioners have often been given little training in how to do this. Their training has largely focused on how to solve presenting problems. Giving advice has formed the basis of most discussions on behaviour change (8). This is despite the evidence that advising people to change aspects of their lifestyles is not very effective, with success rates of only 5–10% (9). Thus, while some patients do seem to respond to advice, most do not. In addition, giving advice can have a negative effect on the relationship between professional and patient or client or customer. It often provokes resistance, with responses such as "Yes, but ..." from the receiver of the advice. Both the health promotion practitioner and the receiver of the advice may be left feeling frustrated and even angry. (It can also, arguably, be criticized as unethical, because it promotes the values of the health promoter, not those of the patient or client.) It is possible to argue that despite the weak effectiveness of this kind of intervention, the benefits of widespread application could nevertheless be considerable. However, now that more effective (and ethical) ways of influencing behaviour are available, continuing to use advice as the primary method cannot be justified.

Helping people to help themselves

The Health Information Service (HIS) is helping people to help themselves. First set up in 1992, as part of the Patient's Charter, it is now linked to a national freephone line (10). Since January 1994 people dialling the freephone number have been linked to their local HIS, funded by their regional health authority. The information provided includes:

- Improving your health.
- Patient's Charter standards.
- Common diseases, conditions and treatments.
- Local self-help groups.
- Local health services.

All these types of health education are likely to be ineffective on their own. They are most effective when they form part of a wider *health promotion* strategy, which includes policies and environments to "back up" the efforts of individual people. So, for example, teaching a patient how to keep a wound clean needs to be backed up by policies and practices which ensure that infections do not spread, whether the transaction with the patient takes place in hospital, in the health centre, in the workplace or in the home. Thus, every one-to-one health education transaction needs to be seen in the wider context of the supports available to the person, which make "healthy choices easier".

UNDERSTANDING YOURSELF AND YOUR CLIENTS (11)

An understanding of how people view themselves and their world is a very useful starting point to help health promoters to change the way they relate to clients. Transactional analysis provides a useful framework for analysing the relationship between health promoter and client (12). Everyone has a basic position from which he or she looks at life, usually largely influenced by their family and the way they were brought up. People can adopt four basic life positions.

"I'm OK—you're OK"

A person adopting this position feels good about themselves and confident in their work ("I'm OK"). They will also feel that in general other people are trustworthy and basically good ("You're OK"). It is a healthy, optimistic and confident position, operating with a belief that people are equal and have equal worth. However, it does not mean looking at life through rose-coloured spectacles, but that people are basically "good enough" despite their quirks and failings.

"I'm OK—you're not OK"

People who take this position are often critical of others and find themselves putting other people down and blaming them. However, people who like doing things for others (rescuing other people) also often have this stance ("You're not OK, so you need me to look after you"). People in this position are likely to have difficulty in learning to trust and rely on others.

"I'm not OK—you're OK"

People with this view will often put themselves down and feel inferior to others. They may feel powerless to change their circumstances and, as a result, get very depressed. People in this position will often discount compliments and praise from other people because "it can't be true because I'm not OK".

"I'm not OK—you're not OK"

People with this view are very vulnerable and may already have chronic health problems such as alcoholism, drug abuse or mental health problems.

Working with them requires an awareness of how the helper can avoid being manipulated into confirming that "not OK" position.

It is important for helpers to work from the "I'm OK, you're OK" position, treating clients as "OK" equals, in order to start the process of helping them to feel more "OK" about themselves, more in control of their lives and therefore better able to make health choices. Using the "I'm OK—you're OK" framework can be useful for identifying some of the stances health and caring professionals and clients may adopt. For example, it is easy for the health promoter to adopt the "I'm OK—you're not OK" position with clients. One version of this is a "persecutor" position, where clients are blamed or criticized. An example is "Yes, but you don't *try* to remember to take your tablets". A more helpful response would be one where the patient is regarded as OK, such as "What would help you to remember to take your tablets?"

The same position of "I'm OK—you're not OK" may also result in the health promoter acting as a "rescuer". "Rescuers" want people to feel better, and to this end they may be falsely reassuring that everything is all right, and try to prevent clients finding out painful things about their situation. In the long term this is harmful, because it confirms that clients are not OK enough to take responsibility for, and control over, their lives. For example, a "rescuer" might say "Let me do it for you. It's easy really", whereas a better response might be "What do you find difficult?" Or a "rescuer" might say "There is no need to get upset. Your little boy will grow out of it", whereas it might be more helpful to say "You're obviously upset about this. Would you like to say more about it?"

Clients who adopt the "I'm not OK" position frequently portray themselves as "victims", thus putting up a barrier against any help the health promoter might offer. For example, a "victim" might say "What do you expect from someone like me? I'm past it at my age." A response which treats this person as OK could be "How much do you think you could still manage?" Another example is "I can't do that. I've never been able to manage the baby. You must think I am stupid." A helpful response, which treats the person as OK, might be "Let's look first at what you *are* managing OK." In these examples the health promoter encourages the "victim" to focus on what *is* OK, on what they *can* do, rather than focusing on what is not OK, which would merely confirm their helpless "victim" position.

I now turn to some of the recent research on influencing people to change their behaviour, which identifies the skills the health promoter requires in order to be able to help effectively.

DEVELOPMENTS IN BEHAVIOURAL RESEARCH

Several developments have taken place in behavioural research over the last 10 years which point to more effective methods of encouraging behaviour change. For example, there is good evidence that the key lies in improving the person's, family's or group's *motivation* to change, and that this can be done by using a negotiation method in which the *patient* or *client* or *family* or *group*, rather than the health promoter, articulates the goals of change, the benefits and costs of change, and the steps towards change. Finding ways of working with people who feel angry, "disempowered", intruded upon, "unmotivated" or resistant is a key issue for all health promoters, whether they are working with individuals or families (where perhaps child abuse or neglect has occurred) or groups of people living in disadvantaged circumstances.

Any model of change must give workers a clear idea about how to work with people who may not want to be worked with. I now describe some of the key features of several models based on recent research. All these models provide a basis for health and social care practitioners to work with people in enabling, rather than disabling, ways.

Solution-focused therapy

This is a model of intervention developed and described by de Shazer and colleagues at the Brief Family Therapy Centre in Milwaukee (13). (It is also referred to as "brief therapy".) It focuses on helping people to discover what solutions or outcomes they desire for their problems, not on the problems themselves. It also stresses the importance of identifying successful behaviours (those which do not have problems) and encouraging clients to repeat and do more of these. Activities that help to enlarge and enhance these behaviours, which are exceptions to the problem, provide the key to the solution. Exceptions are those periods when the expected problem does not occur—for example, when a child who usually has temper tantrums at meal times does not have a tantrum. Solution-focused therapy is goal-driven, but the goals are set by the client, *not* by the "expert" (the doctor or other health or social care practitioner). The role of the facilitator is to help the client to identify realistically achievable goals, and steps towards goals. This is done by asking "change-orientated questions" ("change talk"). One technique is to ask the "miracle question". To do this the facilitator says something like:

> "Suppose there is a miracle and your problems are solved. What will you notice that's different that tells you a miracle has happened?"

The "miracle picture" described by the client is used as a road map to find out what the client wants and for helping the client to identify what might be done to accomplish the desired changes. Using this approach calls for radically different behaviour from practitioners. The "facilitator" (rather than the "expert") is actively engaged in examining the client's experiences, from the client's perspective, looking for change, identifying exceptions, and helping the client to imagine solutions. This done through asking questions which help the client to discover his or her own solutions, and help the client to create a vision of their own preferred future. Some of the key differences between traditional interventions and solution-focused interventions are set out below, and a case example is provided in the following box.

Traditional intervention	*Solution-focused intervention*
The health promoter advises the client and sets goals.	The health promoter helps the client to identify his or her own goals.
The health promoter focuses on problems, as defined *by* the health promoter.	The client and health promoter together focus on exceptions to problems and the desired future.
The benefits and costs of change are defined by the health promoter.	The benefits and costs of change are defined by the client.
The intervention produces resistance.	The intervention produces cooperation.
The intervention reinforces dependence.	The intervention promotes independence.
The intervention uses the resources of the professional.	The intervention builds on the strengths and resources of the clients.

Case example (14)

The following is a conversation between a health visitor and a single teenage mother.

Health visitor: "How did you manage to get yourself up this morning?"

Mother: "I forced myself to get up because the baby was hungry and she was crying."

Health visitor: "I can imagine how tempting it must have been just to have a lie in. What did you do to make yourself get up?"

continued on next page

continued

Mother: "Well I had to. I love my baby and I don't want her to go hungry."

Health visitor: "Is that what keeps you going, that you love your baby?"

Mother: "It's the only thing that keeps me going. I don't want the baby to suffer because of my problems."

Health visitor: "You must love your baby very much. You are a very loving mother, aren't you?"

In this discussion, the health visitor identifies a strength in the mother—that she loves her baby. She then builds on this:

Health visitor: "So what would it take for you to keep on doing this?"

Mother: "I will just have to remember that my baby needs me."

Health visitor: "So what would it take to convince you that you are a good mother?"

Mother: "I'll just have to believe in myself and not listen to people who put me down."

The health visitor is using the desire of the mother to do well by her baby as a motivating force. Once the mother has begun to feel good about herself as a mother, she will begin to find other ways of behaving like a "good mother".

For further information about solution-focused therapy and training available in the UK, see the note at the end of the chapter (15).

The "stages of change" model (16)

One of the most influential concepts to emerge from behavioural research in recent years is that of "readiness to change". It emerged from a model of "the stages of change" developed in North America (17) This model considers change as a process during which people move through a variety of motivational states, and shows how people can best be helped to move from one stage to another. Research shows that strategies based on this model are effective for changing a range of health-related behaviours, such as alcohol and drug abuse, smoking, taking more exercise, weight control and accepting the offer of various types of health screening.

It takes a holistic approach, integrating a range of factors such as the role of personal responsibility and choice, and the impact of social and environmental forces that set very real limits on the individual potential for change. It provides a framework for a wide range of potential interventions by health promoters, as well as describing the process through which individuals go when acting as *their own* agents of change, for example when someone stops smoking without any professional support.

A crucial point is that the process of change can be thought of as a cyclical "revolving door", which people usually go round more than once before emerging into a permanently changed state. It is also important to recognize that some people may never get as far as entering the revolving door.

There are five key stages related to the cycle (18). Research into the behaviour of smokers has established that they do actually move through these stages in a sequential manner:

- *Stage 1—unmotivated*: this is the stage which precedes entry into the change cycle. At this stage a person has no awareness of a need for change, or does not accept it, and no motivation to change habits or lifestyle.
- *Stage 2—undecided*: people at this stage have entered the change cycle but are uncertain or ambivalent about the prospect of change.
- *Stage 3—motivated*: people at this stage are "ready to change"—prepared to change.

Two further stages refer to those people who have already embarked on change:

- *Stage 4—action*: when people enter the "action" stage they actively begin to change the habit.
- *Stage 5—relapse or maintenance*: at this stage people struggle to maintain the change and may experiment with a variety of coping strategies. Although individuals experience the satisfaction of a changed lifestyle for varying amounts of time, most of them cannot exit from the revolving door the first time around. Typically, they relapse back, for example, they start smoking again. Of great importance, however, is that they do not stop there, but move back into the "undecided" stage, engaging in the cycle all over again. Prochaska and Di Clemente have found that on average successful former smokers take three revolutions of change before they find the way to become fully free of the habit, and exit from the revolving door.

By identifying where clients are in the stages of change, health promoters can tailor their interventions to meet individual needs. For example, support with behaviour change, through exploring alternative coping strategies, is appropriate for someone in the "action" or "maintenance" stages. Health education (information giving and awareness raising) is appropriate for someone at the "unmotivated" stage. Techniques to improve motivation are appropriate for someone in the "undecided" stage, and strategies to help people to make decisions are useful for those in the "motivated" (ready to change) stage. Research has shown that only a third of smokers and heavy drinkers are actually ready to change, the rest are in the "unmotivated" or "undecided" stages (19).

Using this model a patient's needs can be assessed and appropriate education or information given, or motivational techniques used, within the constraints of a few minutes' consultation. It may also help to explain why advice giving alone is limited in its effectiveness. If people are not ready to change, they will resist or rebel against advice, resenting the assumption that they are ready to change. It also highlights that actual behaviour change is not the only worthwhile goal to pursue for a brief consultation. Helping somebody to get a clearer view of the outcomes of change, and of the benefits and costs of change, could lead to success at a later point in time. In other words, interventions can be tailored to suit the position which a person is at in the "stages of change", thus ensuring congruence between the agenda of the client and the health promotion practitioner.

The Health Education Board for Scotland has produced a brief intervention package based on these principles (20). Guidelines for general health promotion have also been produced using this model (21). One controlled trial of an intervention based on dividing people into groups ("unmotivated", "undecided" and "motivated") has so far reported its findings (22).

Motivational interviewing

This is a method of facilitating behaviour change which was developed through research on addiction and is based on using counselling skills to guide the negotiation of behaviour change (23). It is appropriate for people who are at the "undecided" or "motivated" (ready to change) stages of change, for example people who are ambivalent about whether they wish to change a particular behaviour: "I want to change, but I don't want to change." Or people who are undecided how best to proceed now that they want to change.

The important thing about motivation is that it belongs to the individual person, but it can be influenced by discussions between health or caring professionals and their patients/clients. Motivational interviewing has three main stages: the goal-setting stage, the information-gathering stage and the negotiation stage.

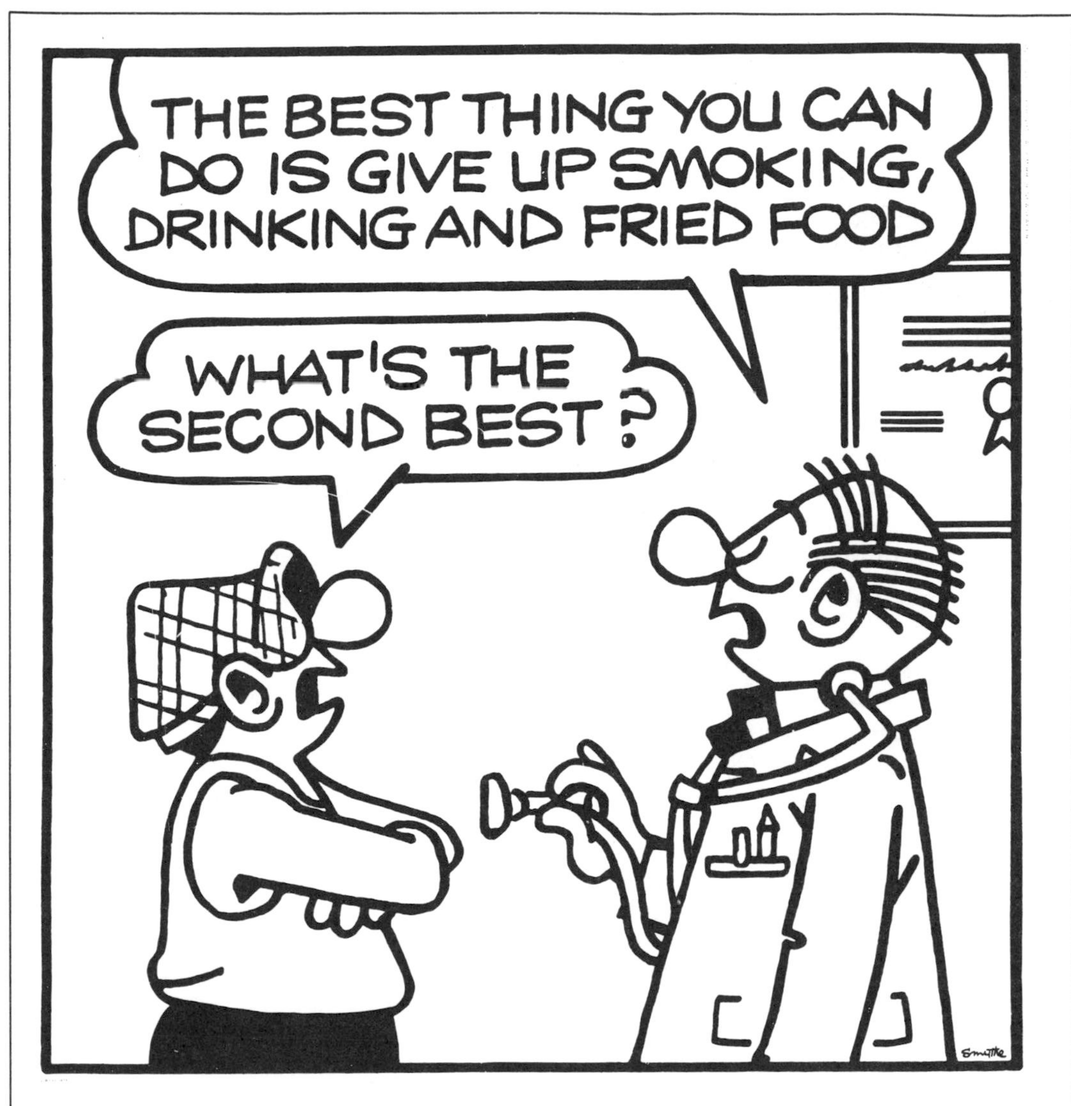

HOW TO LOOK AFTER YOUR HEART.
(A GUIDE FOR PEOPLE WHO ARE ONLY HUMAN.)

Here's some good news. You don't have to become a jogging, teetotal vegetarian to stay young and fit.

There are a few easy changes you can make.

THREE PAINLESS WAYS TO CUT FAT.

1. Cut down on snacks like crisps, biscuits, nibbles.
2. Join the move to skimmed or semi-skimmed milk and low fat spreads.
3. Grill your food instead of frying it.

EXERCISE WITHOUT TEARS.

Try a brisk walk, say twenty minutes or half an hour, three times a week. This will work wonders for your circulation.

THIS BIT'S HARDER (BUT NOT IMPOSSIBLE).

You know that smoking is one of the main causes of heart disease but you don't know how you can possibly survive without a cigarette.

Try giving up for just one day. If you manage that, try again the next day. Join all the ex-smokers who have given up one day at a time.

MAKE A NEW START.

Why be like Andy Capp? Don't forget he is pen and ink but you are flesh and blood.

MAKE A NEW START
LOOK AFTER YOUR HEART!

Figure 9.1 Instead of telling someone what to do, use the model of "the stages of change" to diagnose the person's stage of "readiness to change". Poster reproduced with permission of the Health Education Authority

The goal-setting stage

Start with the person's concerns and help the person to see exactly how they would like things to be different in future. When a person articulates their desired future, they begin to believe in it, and begin to see it as a practical and realizable goal. Get the *patient* to assess the costs and benefits of making the change. Let the patient *persuade you* that they should change, not the other way round.

Techniques which will help include:

- Ask *open* questions: questions which cannot be answered with a "Yes" or "No", or a factual response, but are open to a wide range of answers.
- *Reflect back the concerns of the person*: reflect back the feelings and meanings being expressed by the person. "You are very worried about the way you have put on so much weight recently."
- *Find positive interpretations of the persons abilities*: help the person to "restructure" their view of themselves in order to bolster self-esteem. "I am amazed that you had the will-power to control your drinking for five days. How did you do it?"
- *Act as devil's advocate*: put forward reasons why the person should not change. Skill and good judgement are required about when this is appropriate!
- *Summarize what the person has said*: every few minutes summarize what the person has said and show that you are keen to really understand their situation. Check back that you understand what the person is saying. "So you are worried that your wife will leave you if you don't stop drinking?"

The information-gathering stage

The aim at this stage is to help the person to gather all the information they need in order for them to make a decision and take responsibility for changing their behaviour:

- Provide information; interpret it fairly; answer questions.
- Do not try to prove a point, or persuade the person or give biased information.

The negotiation stage

Focus on what (if anything) the person wants to change, examine options (alternative ways of moving on towards the desired goal), and establish a safe, small, first step.

Many of the basic skills required for effective counselling can be applied to motivational interviewing. For an introduction to the skills of counselling, including its application in helping people to change health behaviours, see Ewles and Simnett (24). For further reading and information about training in counselling, see the note at the end of the chapter (25).

THE FUTURE ROLE OF PRIMARY HEALTH CARE

Primary health care is the point of entry for patients into the treatment, health care and health promotion system. It is vital therefore that secure health promotion foundations are built into primary health care. The elements required to build these foundations are set out in the following box.

The health promotion foundations of primary health care

1. *Influencing local health strategy*: first, all primary health care workers have a key role in contributing to the strategic plans of health commissioners, in order to ensure that these meet the health promotion needs of local people. For example, the health of local homeless people will only be improved when they are provided with adequate shelter; therefore, promoting their health will require health commissioners to commission *housing*. Local authorities and health authorities/health commissions *both* act as health commissioners, and through working together with other local agencies, such as housing associations, they can jointly decide how such needs can best be met, as part of an overall local health strategy. The real needs of local people related to improved health must be addressed and met at local level, whether the need relates to the provision of housing fit for human habitation, employment, healthy working conditions, access to affordable nutritious food, access to affordable leisure and recreational facilities (which may require affordable transport), an unpolluted environment, affordable child care, and many other factors. Primary health care workers must be active in advocating for the health and health promotion needs of their patients, and must ensure that their voice is heard. Local health strategies must be built both bottom-up and top-down, through a foundation on locality (neighbourhood) health strategy evolved in participation with communities.
2. *Purchasing for better health*: second, in future, an increasing number of GPs will have a total fundholding role (26). It is up to them to use this power wisely to meet health promotion and prevention needs—perhaps, for example, to purchase and loan fire-guards to poor families with young children, or to purchase community care for the elderly, mentally

continued on next page

continued

handicapped or those with mental health problems, which will enable them to live healthy lives in the community. GPs will have increasing power to challenge and change established patterns of purchasing, and to ensure a real shift in resources, in order to meet locality prerequisites for health.

3. *Working together for better health*: third, health development through primary health care must become an integral component of locality health promotion strategy and programmes, through primary health care working together with other agencies at a very local level. This will require a clearer definition of health promotion roles and responsibilities, for each member of the primary health care team, so that the work is equitably shared across an "extended primary health care team". For example, GPs have felt that the burden of health behaviour change, and lifestyle change, has been shifted onto them, with the GP contracts (27). A planned "locality" or neighbourhood health promotion strategy should mean that locality policies, programmes, services, projects and all the professions and occupations involved, are working together in each locality, in a concerted way, to the same ends. The role of the GP should be to do what they are best at, in order to contribute effectively to the strategy. This is to assess ("diagnose") the health and health promotion needs of every patient, as an integral part of every consultation, to refer the patient to the appropriate source of health education or health promotion (in addition to medical treatment or medical referral, as required) and to contribute to a review of the progress of both individuals and the whole practice population (i.e., population health gain through treatment and through health promotion) (see Figure 9.2). Thus, in addition to assessing the *health status* of patients (including referral for health checks when necessary), GPs could use the "readiness to change" concept, to assess *the readiness of each patient to change risk behaviours*, and then refer as appropriate.
   - The "unmotivated" could be referred to the receptionist and be given an appropriate health information leaflet, or referred to a health education programme.
   - The "undecided" could be referred for a motivational interview with the practice nurse.
   - The "ready to change" could be referred to an appropriate health promotion service (for example, the local authority fitness advisor for an exercise programme; or the local voluntary agency on alcohol and drugs for help with stopping smoking, taking drugs, or learning how to drink sensibly; or the La Leche league for support with breast feeding).

Increasingly, in future, a wider range of local authority and voluntary organizations will hold regular "health promotion clinics" in the primary health care setting, as part of the extended team. "Health-promoting primary health care centres" will begin to emerge, which place great emphasis on generating a shared sense of purpose, team building, training, personal, professional

continued on next page

continued

and organizational development, quality improvement and multidisciplinary audit of health promotion activities, and on working in partnership with local businesses, schools and other community organizations and people, for better health. The practice business manager will have a key part to play through enabling the development and implemention of the management systems and quality systems which will be required. The whole primary health care team will have a public health (population health gain) orientation and help will be needed from public health medicine specialists and health promotion specialists, to facilitate these developments.

The role of the GP is pivotal to this whole process (which is another example of the operation of the basic health gain cycle) (see Figure 9.2.). Not only does the GP "keep tabs" on the health promotion "career" of each individual patient (with whom a whole range of health promotion

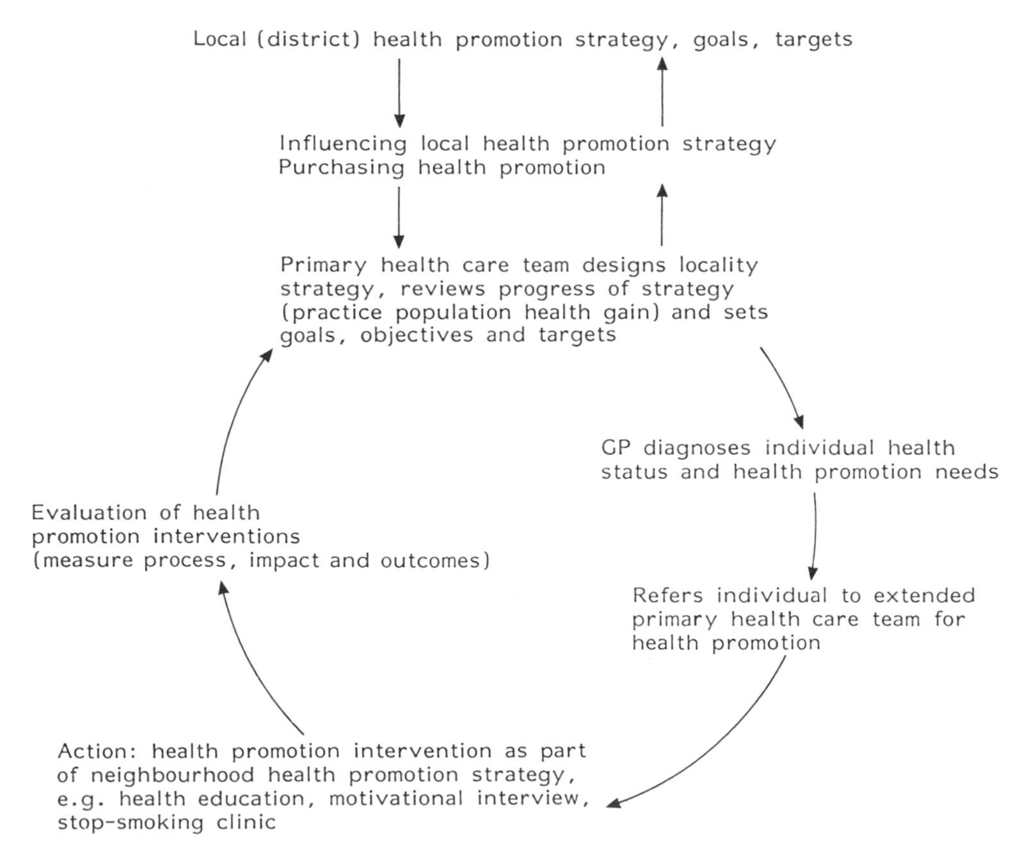

Figure 9.2 The GP as the gateway to health promotion

providers may be involved, from the health service, the local authority, voluntary and commercial agencies, workplaces and beyond), but the GP can use his or her understanding of the health promotion needs of the whole practice population to advocate for these needs to be met in local health-commissioning strategies, and even purchase themselves, to meet these needs, if they are a total fundholding GP. The GP is thus the engine of health gain both through medical diagnosis and health promotion diagnosis, through contributing to the design of the locality (neighbourhood) health promotion strategy, and to the review of progress by the whole primary health care team, and through enabling the provision of an increasing range of treatments, care and health promotion interventions in primary care and community settings. Through the extended primary health care team gaps in health promotion provisions can be plugged, and awareness can be generated about the needs of groups of people who are hard to reach and how to meet them (for example, those living in the neighbourhood who are not registered with a GP).

Federations, or cooperatives, of GP practices are beginning to emerge, based on closer working between locality GP practices and the local community health care trust (28). These are undertaking activities such as locality morbidity-mapping projects to support a community-wide response to *Health of the Nation* targets, and improved peer group support through multidisciplinary education in primary care settings. The Lyme Community Care Unit, set up in 1992, is a general practice-based unit which controls the total health and social care budget for its 8000 population, in return for which its contract with Dorset Health Commission makes it responsible for health gain targets. The unit says it has been able to make savings which have enabled it to expand its health education programmes (29). For training materials, related to the role of GPs in health promotion, see the note at the end of the chapter (30). A recent report from a task group appointed to report to government ministers (published by the NHS Executive) focuses on the future of nursing in primary health care and identifies important keys to nurse development, such as multidisciplinary audit and training in the practice setting, primary health care nursing research, and an extended leadership and management role for nurses in primary health care (31).

DEVELOPING LIFE SKILLS

Opportunities for life skills education exist at all stages in the life cycle. By life skills I mean the key skills necessary for living, such as how to improve self-esteem, how to communicate and relate to others in a morally responsible and "healthy" manner, with respect for oneself and others, and with sensitivity towards the needs and views of others. Learning about how best to live is a continuous process, starting at birth and going on throughout childhood, young adulthood, during working life and at home with the family, and ending with learning how best to die. It should go without saying that these are the most important things we need to learn! Unfortunately, we are often expected to "catch" them automatically, without any proper learning process to help us. To improve on this situation, which arguably is a major contributor to ill-health and human conflicts, such as war and disputes between employers and employees, we need to adopt a "life cycle" strategy, and to introduce appropriate support and learning opportunities at each stage.

One project in Hampshire has made a start by applying this sort of approach to education for parenthood, through the appointment of a development officer to promote initiatives with children and young people, prospective parents and parents (32). This project included the setting up of life skills groups in both primary and secondary schools and at a sixth form college. Unfortunately, though, focusing life skills education on parenthood can lead to the exclusion of boys and young men. In fact, these same life skills are needed to relate to others in a very wide range of situations, and through taking a broader approach it may be possible to find new opportunities for learning them.

- The National Curriculum obliges schools to provide a broad and balanced curriculum which must "prepare pupils for the opportunities, responsibilities and experiences of adult life" (33). This will require schools to give high priority to the cross-curricular themes of education for citizenship and health education. Further adjustments are needed following the Dearing review (34). A Health Education Authority survey (35) has emphasized that some of the ground gained in the early 1980s is in danger of being lost, and that the targets set in *The Health of the Nation*, especially those related to a reduction in the number of teenage pregnancies, and to reductions in smoking and drug use in young people, will not be achieved without high-quality school-based health education. Useful resources have been developed for use with young people (36).
- Opportunities for life skills education also exist beyond and outside school. The workplace is a source of untapped potential, through developing the potential of staff and managers to work together to improve performance and the quality of working life, through improved relationships and communication. As a result of a project to study stress in the staff of Northumberland Health Authority, and the

finding that staff in four out of five directorates reported relationships with other people as their greatest source of stress, the Health Authority is setting up groups to explore the nature and extent of relationship difficulties and to discuss how improvements could be made (37). The development of "quality improvement" (including audit) health promotion training in workplaces will be another step in the right direction. Adult and continuing education provisions make a valuable contribution but tend not to reach those in greatest need.

- One way to develop these life skills is to choose relationships with people who are healthier than you, and to choose to work for healthy organizations (i.e., to select healthy "models"). This option may not be open to everyone, but many people do, in fact, choose it. There is a body of recent research on the characteristics of the most healthy people (38). One notable characteristic of the most healthy people is that they tend not to be interested in power for its own sake, but are concerned to share it as far as possible and to empower other members of society. Choose your partners and mentors in life very carefully!
- One thing we can all do is to concentrate less on changing other people, and more on developing ourselves.

For further reading on life skills, see the note at the end of the chapter (39).

REACHING THE PARTS AND PEOPLE THAT OTHERS MISS

I now turn to a very important issue for health promotion: how do we involve those groups of people who are hard to reach, such as the homeless, the mentally ill, the unemployed and the poor, who may be the groups with the greatest needs? One effective way is through advocacy schemes. *Advocacy* is generally taken to mean representing the interests of people who cannot speak up for themselves. However, in health promotion terms, it involves more than this. It is concerned with using every possible means to assist people to become independent and *self-advocating*. Recent research has established the effectiveness, for example, of bilingual advocacy schemes (40) These schemes are very diverse, and a positive feature of this diversity is that it offers different routes for non-English-speaking communities into a better understanding of their health and into the confidence and empowerment necessary for taking increased control over their own health. However, existing advocacy schemes only cover a small proportion of existing need, and the challenge for purchasers and providers is the scale of the unmet need and how resources can be found to meet these needs.

Community-based work is a way of reaching hard-to-reach groups (41). Going into disadvantaged and poor communities with an imposed agenda of lifestyle issues such as smoking, diet, exercise and so on will not be successful because there may be other issues which are much more pressing on people's lives. So, it is crucial to start by identifying the issues which are important to the residents themselves, and to adopt an approach based on community empowerment through:

- Developing perceptions of self-esteem and self-worth.
- Mobilizing people in existing community groups to build on their own strengths and resources.
- Enabling the community to make real improvements in environmental and health conditions.
- Enabling people to experience a sense of community and increased control over their own destiny.

One recent successful project provides guidance about how this can be done.

Bournville Community Development Project (42)

The Bournville is a deprived housing estate in Weston-super-Mare. A community heart disease prevention project between 1991 and 1993 was a national demonstration project mounted by Look after Your Heart–Avon. It evolved a system of tracking progress by recording changes in specific areas, through an outcomes measures checklist, such as:

- Participation rates in health-related action.
- Perceived changes in knowledge, attitudes and behaviour of specific subgroups of the population.
- Changes in the availability of health-promoting facilities and resources (such as exercise groups and facilities, and support groups for parents).

The evaluation indicates eight key ingredients for success:

1. *The community empowerment approach*: the project did not start with an imposed "top-down" agenda of heart health risk factors, but started by responding to the issues which local people saw as most important to them.
2. *The project worker*: the project worker was accessible, with an office on the estate, semi-autonomous, with control of a small budget, highly competent in the skills and attitudes required for community work, and "knew the ropes" about how statutory organizations work.
3. *The local and national agencies*: the sustained commitment of the agencies in LAYH–Avon, and the HEA, over a period of five years, was vital.

continued on next page

continued

4. *Networks*: well-established networks at all levels, from fieldworkers to chief executives, chairpersons and politicians, were vital.
5. *Support on the ground*: support for the project worker from local agencies and local people.
6. *High profile*: media publicity and reports to statutory agencies helped to sustain the project.
7. *Evaluation process*: a structured evaluation process demonstrated that tangible results were being achieved.
8. *Planning for the end*: embedding developments in the permanent structures of statutory agencies gained long-term commitment to the Bournville and its residents.

The major achievements of the project included new facilities and groups for mothers and young children, setting up a needle exchange scheme at the estate chemist shop, the establishment of a community newspaper, opening a multi-purpose health and social services locality centre where activities focused on health and social well-being take place, and environmental improvements such as new playgrounds and a new pelican crossing.

More important, though, than these tangible changes is the changed climate: the Bournville is now a happy place with people who feel that life is worthwhile and who want to live life to the full.

CONCLUDING THOUGHTS

At the heart of health promotion are relationships. In the end, the bottom line for effective health promotion lies in the nature of these relationships—whether they are mutually empowering, so that the self-esteem and well-being of everyone is improved. Improving these relationships will require big efforts across all the organizations and groups which contribute to the infrastructure of our society: families, community groups, hospitals, schools, businesses, the criminal justice system, the media, and all public sector services. To do this we need to become a learning society, focused not on the problems of the present, but on the healthier and more satisfying future which lies within our grasp.

Achieving these healthier relationships cannot be done by just focusing on improving the relationships of the individuals concerned. It needs the back-up of all the organizations contributing to a community, through creating a climate, systems, structures and processes which truly empower local people to look after their own, and others', well-being. This book has described how to set about doing it. The life-blood of health development is enhanced communication, so that best practices spread, innovations are encouraged, mistakes become learning opportunities, and working together becomes a truly integrated process. Hierarchical organizations stifle communication, so we must develop flatter organizations, based on the work of semi-autonomous teams. Developing health-promoting communities is not a mirage or a dream: we have much of the knowledge required and successful models to build on. I hope that this book will make a contribution to progress.

If this book has done nothing else, I hope that it has at least improved your vision of what this healthier future could be like. Better still, I hope that you have identified some small, safe steps which you could take (with support), to help to make it a reality.

An activity you could undertake: Learning from mistakes

Think of one specific mistake which was recently made by a particular person in your organization. Analyse what happened through describing:

1. The *antecedents*: the situation before the mistake occurred: the culture of the organization about how to deal with mistakes, stress levels in the particular department or team, factors related to the individual concerned.
2. The *behaviour of those involved when the mistake occurred*—describe the behaviour of the key people involved.
3. The *consequences*—what were the outcomes for the person who made the mistake, for the key people involved, and for the organization as a whole? Were these outcomes desirable or undesirable? (For example, will they prevent further mistakes occurring? Was the person who made the mistake deliberately humiliated? Was the damage to the victims of the mistake repaired? Was the team or organization able to learn from the mistake?)

Can you now think of anything which could have been done differently, in order to improve the outcomes for the person who made the mistake, for the key people involved, for the victims of the mistake, or for the organization as a whole?

NOTES, REFERENCES AND FURTHER READING

(1) For a discussion on the ineffectiveness of most communication, and of the skills required to bridge the "interpersonal gap", see:

Bolton, R. (1979) *People Skills*. Englewood Cliffs, NJ: Prentice-Hall.

(2) For a very readable and research-based account of what makes healthy individuals, families, workplaces, organizations and societies, see:

Skynner, R. and Cleese, J. (1993) *Life and How to Survive It*. London: Methuen.

(3) Woolf, H., Tumin, S. and Faulkner, D. (1994) *Relational Justice: Repairing The Breach*. Winchester: Waterside Press.

(4) Reported by David Brindle in *The Guardian*, 7 December 1994, p. 8.

(5) A full exploration of the argument that health professionals undermine people's own ability to cope is found in:

Illich, I. (1977) *Limits to Medicine*. Harmondsworth: Pelican.

For a shorter account of this argument, see:

Illich, I. (1978) Medical nemesis. In Tucket, D. and Kaufert, J. (eds), *Basic Readings in Medical Sociology*. London: Tavistock. Ch. 29.

For a general discussion on the relevance of sociology for health promotion, and of the need for health promoters to ask key sociological questions, such as "In whose interests is this?" "How is power being exercised?" "Whose values are being prioritized?" see the contribution by Nicki Thorogood in:

Bunton, R. and Macdonald, G. (eds) (1992) *Health Promotion: Disciplines and Diversity*. London: Routledge. Ch. 3.

(6) Weare, K. (1992) The contribution of education to health promotion. In Bunton, R. and Macdonald, G. (eds), *Health Promotion: Disciplines and Diversity*. London: Routledge. Ch. 4.

(7) Hart, J.T. (1988) *A New Kind of Doctor*. London: Merlin Press.

(8) See, for example:

Tuckett, D., Boulton, M., Olson, C. and Williams, A. (1985) *Meetings Between Experts: An Approach to Sharing Ideas in Medical Consultations*. London: Tavistock.

Russell, M., Wilson, C., Baker, C. and Taylor, C. (1979) Effect of general practitioners' advice against smoking. British Medical Journal, **ii**, 231–235.

(9) See, for example:

Kottke, T. and Battista, R.N. (1988) Attributes of successful smoking interventions in medical practice: a meta analysis of 39 controlled trials. *Journal of the American Medical Association* **259**: 2882–2889.

(10) Freephone 0800 66 55 44. To find out more about the Health Information Service (HIS), write to Amanda Arrowsmith, Patient Empowerment Unit, NHS Executive, Headquarters, Room 4N34B, Quarry House, Quarry Hill, Leeds LS2 7UE.

(11) This section is based on a discussion in:

Ewles, L. and Simnett, I. (lst edn, 1985) *Promoting Health: A Practical Guide to Health Education*. Chichester: Wiley. Ch. 9.

(12) For further reading on transactional analysis, see:

Harris, T.A (1973) *I'm OK, You're OK*. Harmondsworth: Pan.

Harris, T.A. and Harris, A.B. (1986) *Staying OK*. London: Pan.

Berne, E. (1964) *Games People Play*. Harmondsworth: Pan.

(13) See:

de Shazer, S. (1991) *Putting Difference to Work*. New York: Norton.

(14) This case example is based on information in:

Berg, I.K. (1991) *Family Preservation: A Brief Therapy Workbook*. London: Brief Therapy Press.

For further information on brief therapy practice in the UK, see:

George, E., Iveson, C and Ratner H. (1990) *Problem to Solution: Brief Therapy with Individuals and Families*. London: Brief Therapy Press.

For information about the availability of Brief Therapy Press publications, and about brief therapy training available in the UK, see note (11) in Chapter 4.

(15) For an easily understood UK publication, and for information about training, see note (11) in Chapter 4.

(16) For information about the availability of "train the trainers" courses in the use of this model, contact the "Helping People Change" Project Coordinator, HEA Primary Health Care Unit, Block 10, Churchill Hospital, Headington, Oxford OX3 7LJ. Telephone: 01865 226045. These courses provide professionals with booklets of guidelines to support them in their work, and with self-help booklets to use with patients/clients wishing to change a particular behaviour.

(17) Prochaska, J.O. and Di Clemente C.C. (1982) Transtheoretical therapy: towards a more integrative model of change. *Psychotherapy*: Theory, *Research and Practice* **19** (3): 276–288.

Prochaska J. and Di Clemente C. (1984) *The Transtheoretical Approach: Crossing Traditional Boundaries of Therapy*. Harnewood, Illinois: Dow-Jones-Homewood.

The Health Education Authority Primary Health Care Unit at Oxford, established in 1989, has assisted delivery of health education in primary health care through its programme of team workshops, publications and research, and through the national facilitator network. This includes a "Helping People Change" project based on "The Stages of Change" model. For further information, see note (16).

The "Get Moving" project in Bristol is evaluating how GPs and practice nurses can help patients to take more physical activity, through a controlled trial using an adapted version of the Prochaska and Di Clemente model. This is a joint initiative between a multi-agency heart disease prevention programme "Look After Your Heart—Avon" and Bristol University. For further information contact the Team Manager for Heart Health, Bristol Area Specialist Health Promotion Service, Southmead Hospital, Westbury on Trym, Bristol BS10 5NB. Telephone: 0117 9505 050.

(18) For further information on this model, see:

Ewles, L. and Simnett, I. (3rd edn, 1995) *Promoting Health: A Practical Guide.* London: Scutari Press. Ch. 10.

(19) Rollnick, S., Heather, N., Gold, R. and Hall, W. (1992) Development of a short "readiness to change" questionnaire for use in brief opportunistic interventions among excessive drinkers. *British Journal of Addiction* **87**: 743–754.

Rollnick, S., Kinnersley, P. and Stott, N. (1993) Methods of helping patients with behaviour change. *British Medical Journal* **307**, 188–190.

(20) Health Education Board for Scotland (1991) *Drinking Reasonably and Moderately with Self-control (DRAMS)*. Edinburgh: HEBS.

(21) Field, J. and Henderson, J. (1993) *Better Living Better Life*. Henley on Thames: Knowledge House.

(22) Heather, N., Campion, P., Neville, R. and Maccabe, D. (1987) Evaluation of a controlled drinking minimal intervention for problem drinkers in general practice. *Journal of the Royal College of General Practitioners* **37**: 358–363.

(23) A technique useful in the "undecided" stage of change is "motivational interviewing". The emphasis is on exploring a client's concerns, in order to help them move to the "motivated" stage when they are ready to do so. For more information on motivational interviewing, see:

Miller W. and Rollnick S. (1991) *Motivational Interviewing: Preparing People for Change.* Guilford Press: New York.

Rollnick S., Heather N. and Bell, A. (1992) Negotiating behaviour change in medical settings: the development of brief motivational interviewing. *Journal of Mental Health* **1**: 25–37.

(24) Ewles, L. and Simnett, I. (3rd edn, 1995) *Promoting Health: A Practical Guide.* London: Scutari Press. Ch. 10.

(25) For further reading on counselling, see:

Dass, R. and Gorman, P. (1985) *How Can I Help?* London: Rider.

Nelson-Jones, R. (2nd edn, 1988) *Practical Counselling and Helping Skills: Helping Clients to Help Themselves.* London: Cassell Educational.

The Scottish Health Education Group (SHEG), now the Health Education Board for Scotland (HEBS). have produced a guide for those wishing to set up and run short introductory counselling courses for nurses, midwives and health visitors:

SHEG (1990) *Sharing Counselling Skills: A Guide to Running Courses for Nurses, Midwives and Health Visitors.* Available from HEBS, Woodburn House, Canaan Lane, Edinburgh EH10 4SG.

SHEG have also produced a series of six modular courses in counselling and helping skills, which are designed to be used separately or in combination:

Carruthers, T. (1991) *Initial Interviewing and Assessment Skills.* Edinburgh: SHEG.

Woolfe, R. (1991) *Counselling Skills: A Training Manual*. Edinburgh: SHEG.

Robinson, F. and Robson, K. (1991) *Problem Identification and Personal Problem Solving*. Edinburgh: SHEG.

Woolfe, R. and Fewell, J. (1991) *Groupwork Skills: An Introduction*. Edinburgh: SHEG.

Evison, R. (1991) *Personal and Intra-agency Support and Supervision*. Edinburgh: SHEG.

Cherry, C., Robertson, N. and Meadows, F. (1991) *Personal and Professional Development for Group Leaders*. Edinburgh: SHEG.

See also:

SHEG (1989) *HIV/AIDS: Counselling Skills for the General Practitioner*. A videotape plus training notes, available from HEBS (address above).

(26) For detailed discussion of proposals for a major expansion of GP fundholding, see:

NHS Executive (1994) *Developing NHS Purchasing and GP Fundholding: Towards a Primary Care-led NHS*. London: Department of Health.

For a copy of this publication write to Health Publications Unit, DSS Distribution Centre, Heywood Stores, Manchester Road, Heywood, Lancs LO10 2PZ.

(27) Mant, D. (1994) Prevention: primary care tomorrow. *Lancet* 344: 1343–1346.

(28) See, for example:

Sloane, R. (1994) Open for business. *Health Service Journal* 104 (5432): 36.

(29) For further information, contact Lyme community care unit. Telephone: 01297 442254.

(30) Useful resources for use within primary care are:

- A multi-disciplinary training programme for primary health care teams, with a package of materials (course notes, a manual on risk factor management, a detailed practice guide on screening techniques and a resource pack of reference material) available from Radcliffe Medical Press Ltd, 15 Kings Meadow, Ferry Hinksey Road, Oxford OX2 ODP. Telephone: 01865 790696.
- Training packs from Anticipatory Care In Practice, Radcliffe Infirmary, Woodstock Road Oxford OX2 6HE.

(31) NHS Management Executive (1993) *Nursing in Primary Health Care: New World, New Opportunities*. London: HMSO.

(32) Pugh, G. and Poulton, L. (1987) *Parenting as a Job for Life*. London: National Children's Bureau.

For a review of Education for Parenthood and Family Life, see *Highlight* No. 130 (1994). *Highlight* is a regular information sheet produced by the National

Children's Bureau, 8 Wakley Street, London, EC1V 7QE. Telephone: 0171 843 6000.

(33) Department of Education and Science (1988) *The Education Reform Act 1988*. London: HMSO.

(34) Dearing, R. (1994) *The National Curriculum and Its Assessment: Final Report*. School Curriculum and Assessment Authority.

(35) National Foundation for Educational Research (1993) *A Survey of Health Education Policies in Schools*. London: Health Education Authority.

(36) Hopson, B. and Scally, M. (1979–1988) *Life Skills Teaching Programmes Manuals 1, 2, 3 and 4*. Leeds: Lifeskills Associates. Available from Lifeskills Associates, Ashling, Back Church Lane, Leeds LS16 8DN.

TACADE (1986) *Skills for Adolescence: A programme for Age 11–14*. Salford: TACADE and Quest International. For information about the availability of TACADE publications, see note (23) in Chapter 8.

Living Skills 1 (1987) London: Boulton Hawker.

Living Skills 2 (1994) St. Leonards on Sea, East Sussex: Outset Publishing. Available from Outset Publishing, Conqueror Industrial Estate, Moorhurst Road, St Leonards on Sea, East Sussex TN38 9NA.

Gray, G. and Hill, F. (1987) *Health Action Pack: Health Education for 16–19s*. Cambridge: National Extension College.

Anderson, J. (1988) *Health Skills Training Manual*. London: Health Education Authority.

Clarity Collective (1988) *Taught not Caught*. Cambridge: Learning Development Aids.

Health Education Authority (1989) *Health for Life: The Health Education Authority Primary School Project*. Walton-on-Thames: Nelson.

Health Education Board for Scotland (1994) *Promoting the Health of Young People in Europe: A Training Manual*. Edinburgh: Health Education Board for Scotland.

(37) Paxton, R. and Axelby, J. (1994) Is Stress Your Occupation? *Health Service Journal* **104** (5428): 30–31.

(38) See:

Skynner, R. and Cleese, J. (1993) *Life and How to Survive It*. London: Methuen. Ch 1.

Beavers, R. (1990) *Successful Families*. New York: Norton.

(39) Burnard, P. (1985) *Learning Human Skills: A Guide for Nurses*. Oxford: Heinemann Nursing.

Skynner, R. and Cleese, J. (1984) *Families and How to Survive Them*. London: Methuen.

Bolton. R. (1979) *People Skills*. Englewood Cliffs, NJ: Prentice Hall.

Honey, P. (1980) *Solving People Problems*. Maidenhead, Berks: McGraw-Hill.

Gordon, T. (1976) *Parent Effectiveness Training in Action*. New York: Perigee Books.

Adams, L. with Lenz, E. (1979) *Effectiveness Training for Women*. New York: Perigee Books.

Cox, G. and Dainow, S. (1985) *Making the Most of Yourself*. London: Fontana.

Pedlar, M and Boydell, T. (1985) *Managing Yourself*. London: Fontana.

Thorne, M. and Fritchie, R. (1985) *Interpersonal Skills for Women Managers: a Tutor's Guide*. Bristol: MSC Training Services/Bristol Polytechnic.

Francis, D. and Woodcock, M. (1982) *Fifty Activities for Self-development*. Aldershot: Gower.

Nelson-Jones, R. (1986) *Human Relationship Skills: Training and Self-help*. Eastbourne: Cassell.

(40) Parsons, L. and Rudat, K. (1994) The power of advocacy. *Health Service Journal*, **104** (5429): 31.

(41) By community-based health promotion work, I mean work that directly involves health promoters in working with groups of the public in a sustained way which enables them to increase control over, and improve, their health. It includes community development work, community outreach schemes, advocacy schemes and self-help groups.

For a detailed discussion on how best to work with communities, see:

Ewles, L. and Simnett, I. (3rd edn, 1995) *Promoting Health: A Practical Guide*. London: Scutari Press. Ch. 12.

For training materials on community-based work, see:

Johnston, M.P. and Rifkin, S.B. (eds) (1987) *Health Care Together: Training Exercises for Health Workers in Community-based Programmes*. London: Macmillan/Teaching Aids at Low Cost.

For a North American text on community-based health promotion work, see:

Bracht, N. (ed.) (1990) *Health Promotion at the Community Level*. Newbury Park, CA: Sage Sourcebooks for the Human Services Series 15.

(42) This case study is based on the report of a community heart disease prevention project on the Bournville estate, Weston-super-Mare, Avon, which took place between 1991 and 1993. The project was undertaken by *Look After Your Heart—Avon* (LAYH—Avon) with help through funding from a Health Education Authority award. For a copy of the report, contact Look After Your Heart-Avon, Bristol Area Specialist Health Promotion Service, Frenchay Healthcare NHS Trust, Beckspool Road, Frenchay, Bristol BS16 1ND. Telephone: 0117 9701 212.

INDEX

Index compiled by Campbell Purton

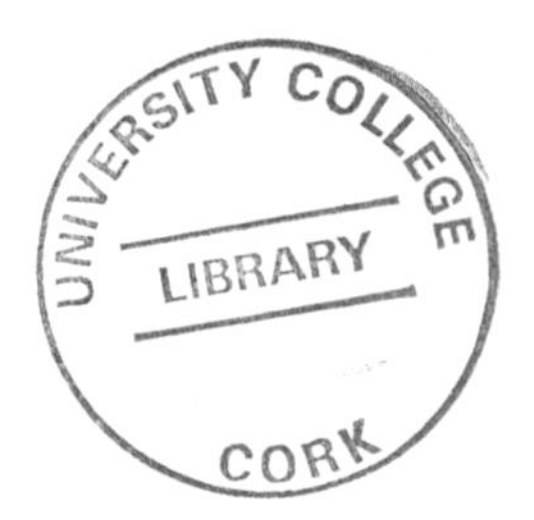